From Stethoscope to Boardroom

Chief Medical Officer Decoded

BELA NAND, MD, MBA

Ballast Books, LLC
www.ballastbooks.com

ISBNs:
Hardcover: 978-1-971678-13-9
Paperback: 978-1-971678-14-6

Printed in the United States of America

Published by Ballast Books
www.ballastbooks.com

For more information, bulk orders, appearances, or speaking requests, please email: info@ballastbooks.com

CONTENTS

FOREWORD

by
Jeffrey Kuhlman, MD

Some lessons arrive quietly, long before we recognize how profoundly they will shape us. I can still remember my very first day of medical school. I was a nineteen-year-old sitting in an amphitheater, taking in the simple but foundational truths the dean laid out before us:

1. Listen to your patients. They will tell you what is wrong with them.
2. Don't become overenamored with technology.
3. Give every patient something during their time of need.

At the time, I thought these were clinical pearls. With experience, I realized they were leadership principles—ones that would accompany me through thirty years in the US Navy, through deployments, through caring for the president of the United States, through serving as the chief medical officer of the nation's largest hospital, and now through my work guiding quality and safety across a national health system. Those lessons have been my compass, and they came back to me as I read *From Stethoscope to Boardroom*.

Dr. Bela Nand has written a book that speaks directly to the heart of what it means to lead as a physician. Her insights remind me of the countless transitions we undergo in our careers—from novice to expert, from clinician to leader, from individual contributor to steward of systems and people. She captures the emotional, intellectual, and moral challenges of that evolution with honesty and clarity.

During my three decades in uniform, I learned that leadership is never about rank. It is about responsibility—to your mission, your team, and the people you serve. I saw young corpsmen in their twenties perform with the composure of seasoned officers. I witnessed teams make life-and-death decisions in austere environments where protocols mattered, but character mattered more. I learned that the best leaders are those who listen first, speak with purpose, and act with integrity—the very themes woven through this manuscript.

What struck me as I read this book is how deeply Dr. Nand understands the real, unvarnished work of a chief medical officer. The CMO role is not glamorous. It is not about titles or visibility or accolades. It is about influence without authority, accountability without always having the levers you wish you had, and the constant challenge of translating organizational priorities into clinical realities. It is also, as she rightly points out, a profoundly human role.

Whether in the Situation Room, an aircraft carrier, the Oval Office, or the largest hospital in the nation, I have learned that leadership is not defined by the scale of the environment but by the weight of the moments: The late-night calls after an adverse event. The conversations with physicians after a near miss. The family you meet at their most vulnerable hour. The nurse who needs reassurance. The resident who needs honesty. The senior surgeon who needs someone to tell him the truth with respect. These are the moments that test us and ultimately shape us.

Dr. Nand captures all of this with precision and empathy. She reminds us that physicians entering leadership must grow in ways that extend far beyond clinical mastery. Emotional intelligence, humility, courage, the ability to create psychological safety—these are not soft skills. They are mission critical. They are what keep teams functioning during crises. They are what sustain organizations through change. They are what protect patients when systems fail.

What I appreciate even more is her message to aspiring physician leaders: “You are needed now more than ever.” Health care is in the midst of accelerated transformation—technological, financial, cultural, and ethical. We cannot afford for our most thoughtful, compassionate, and resilient physicians to sit on the sidelines. We need their voices in the boardroom, their discernment in strategy, their integrity in decision-making, and their unwavering commitment to the patient at the center of it all.

For those considering this journey, this book will serve as a guide and a grounding point. For those already in the arena, it will feel like a conversation with a trusted colleague who understands the pressures, the doubts, and the quiet victories. And for every physician who has ever felt the tension between clinical identity and administrative responsibility, it will offer both clarity and courage.

As I reflect on my own career—from medical school to US Navy service, from the West Wing to the largest hospital in America, and now across a national health system—I am reminded that the essence of our work has never changed:

Listen deeply.

Stay grounded in what truly matters.

Give something meaningful to every person who crosses your path.

Dr. Nand’s book not only reaffirms these truths—it extends them into the future of health care leadership.

It is my privilege to contribute this foreword and to recommend this book to every physician who feels called to lead. Your journey will be demanding. It will stretch you. It will change you. But if you lead with purpose, humility, and heart, it will also be the most meaningful work you ever do. The purpose of life is to live a life of purpose.

—Jeffrey Kuhlman, MD, MPH
Captain, Medical Corps, US Navy (Ret.)
Chief quality and safety officer, AdventHealth
Chief medical officer, Florida Hospital, 2013–2019
White House physician, 2000–2013

Introduction

SO, YOU MIGHT WANT TO BE A CHIEF MEDICAL OFFICER?

The chief medical officer (CMO) is the strongest and loudest voice supporting quality and patient safety in any health care organization. It is also the only C-suite role that, by design, crosses the chasm between the clinical and administrative wings. To be effective in this role, physician leaders must learn how to influence rather than merely command. They need to find ways to reduce or remove friction between departments.

For that reason, I think of the CMO as a health care organization's relational WD-40. And not all physicians can lead in this way! This role can be both exciting and frustrating at the same time; it depends on which day you ask.

This book offers my perspective on the key training, experience, personality traits, and learned competencies required to succeed as a CMO. It is designed to help physician executives learn what to expect when exploring this role as a possible future career path. I also want to enable health care organizations to understand what to look for in a CMO candidate and to encourage them to explore an expanded role for the CMO, one that can strengthen an entire operation. The question posed most often these days by health care organizations is not *why* they need a CMO, but *how* they can leverage the role for the benefit of the patients whom we are so privileged to serve as health care leaders.

To help set the stage for what lies ahead, I'd like you to consider what a "typical" day as a CMO might look like for you.

A "Typical" Day for a CMO

No sooner do you sit at your desk to begin your day at an ungodly early morning hour than the CEO requests that you speak with a certain physician regarding some transfers. Disagreements on that issue have caused several ongoing problems, and he wants you to head them off before they become serious.

Not more than fifteen minutes later, the chief nursing officer flies into your office, almost breathless. She hurriedly describes an unpleasant incident that just occurred, *again*, with a seasoned and talented but crusty surgeon. "Would you please intervene?" she pleads.

Later that morning, the director of quality seeks you out to report that the hospital's CAUTI numbers are increasing. "Could you investigate to see what's causing the increase?" he asks.

As you tackle that problem, the director of radiology reports to you that the CT machine is down. "Should we go on bypass?" she wonders aloud.

You have barely enough time to take a breath before your phone rings. It's the medical staff president, calling to ask about the hospital's communication plan. You talk through its current status and hang up the phone . . . and then you notice that lunch is still well over an hour away.

This is a typical day? *Really?* Yes, really.

To make the situation even more challenging, keep in mind that although *none* of these departments or individuals report to you, they *all* expect quick answers from you. In that kind of pressure cooker, how can you make good things consistently happen?

Perhaps the most effective and best way to do so is by forging and maintaining strong relationships throughout the organization. Such relationships help you to decrease friction between multiple players. Don't forget, *you're* the organization's relational WD-40.

Does that sound easy? If you think so, imagine what it's like to try to persuade multiple type A personalities to reach a consensus regarding a major change to a process that's been in place for more than a decade. What kind of individual can quickly lay the foundation for such a new and unfamiliar structure? Or perhaps more to the point, who in their right mind would even want to *try*? It takes a special kind of individual to answer, "Well, *I* would."

Do you think *you* could be that special kind of individual? If so, then I believe this book can provide you with seasoned counsel, helpful suggestions, and even "homework" designed to help make your pursuit both encouraging and successful. But let me be clear: This role is not for the faint of heart!

A Changing Role

The role of the chief medical officer has markedly evolved over the past decade. Although job descriptions are becoming more defined in the industry, they still vary widely and can be ambiguous across institutions. In general, this role collaborates with all departments to help institutions achieve the Quadruple Aim of delivering high-quality and efficient care with maximum satisfaction for both patients and associates.

Despite growing curiosity about this role across all disciplines of health care, relatively little literature exists on the topic. What does the role of a CMO entail? Who makes an effective CMO? What should hospitals look for when they hire someone for this position? Do most physicians grasp what the role does? How can female physician leaders prepare themselves for the special challenges that many of them are likely to face? What core competencies are required to effectively execute this role? How does a talented CMO positively impact the health care institution, its medical staff, and the patients it serves?

By contrast, *many* articles have been published in the past few years regarding how to be an effective physician leader and how to train physicians to tackle that challenging role. These articles discuss the key differences regarding the core competencies of physicians versus physician leaders, as well as methods for improving these core competencies and adjusting modern leadership styles to align with traditional practices.

Unfortunately, little information published to date discusses how to harness a physician's inherent style for everyone's benefit. This book addresses that deficit in a very practical, encouraging way. It does so, in part, by including the voices and experiences of many other health care professionals whose jobs intersect with the CMO's at various points. In *From Stethoscope to Boardroom*, you'll hear from experts serving in the roles of chief executive officer, chief operating officer, chief financial officer, chief nursing officer, and more, who suggest from their own viewpoints how CMOs can form good working partnerships designed to benefit both the patients and members of an organization.

This book is *not* about general leadership principles that may apply to anyone seeking some kind of leadership role in the field of medicine. Rather, it aims to answer specific questions pertaining to the crucial role of a CMO serving in an acute care hospital or other health care organization. It provides clear and helpful guidance on the hiring and development of new CMOs, and it also offers aspiring physicians practical advice on how to effectively pursue the role, grow in it, and become more marketable for it.

If you feel that this is your calling, then this book will give you the tools to lead with purpose and confidence.

A Unique and Challenging Position

The chief medical officer position is unique and challenging in the executive suite, as CMOs must work hard to maintain a balance between the concerns of medical staff and those of business administrators.

In my experience, most physicians like to cut to the chase and avoid meetings. They reason, *Why meet when I already know the solution? It's so obvious!* They do so not realizing that the solution they are proposing may work for *their* patient or department, but it might not be the right answer for another.

To be effective in this complex role, the CMO must learn how to interact with and influence various departments whose members do not directly report to them. A CMO must therefore look at the bigger picture and explore possible solutions within the context of a community rather than an individual. This happens most fruitfully when the individuals involved can gain common ground, which is most often achieved when a CMO exercises their hard-won influence in an environment where everyone has the freedom to clearly share their differing visions.

Effective CMOs must strategically develop a *team* of future physician leaders who learn to use their talents for the betterment of the community at large. This is hard work, made more difficult because the authoritative or pyramidal/hierarchical nature of medicine still exists. It is the role of the CMO to change this pyramid into a square toolbox in which everyone works in tandem to achieve the same goal: high-quality, safe care for patients.

The return on investment (ROI) for this role is simple yet complicated. Hospital metrics such as length of stay (LOS), readmission rate, and patient experience are easily measured. A wide range of dashboards is available for each of these purposes and more.

An equally important ROI is culture alignment, which is incalculable. How can a CMO move the medical staff and hospital administration in the same direction, decrease burnout for physicians, and develop long-term growth for physician leaders—all at the same time?

In my view, the biggest bang for the buck for the CMO role comes in delivering high-quality care and excellent patient safety. In a very real sense, this is the *only* product for any health care system. If the product is poor, the market will reject it and the hospital will close shop. *Everything* follows quality—and no one is more qualified to build a high-quality product than an effective CMO.

Purpose and Audience

In this book, I want to showcase how underutilized yet important the CMO is in the C-suite of any health care organization. I have in mind not only acute hospitals (where I currently work), but also insurance companies, post-acute facilities, and many other organizations.

My primary audience is physicians who aspire to serve in this role. It is essential that they recognize how to prepare effectively and that they determine the most strategic areas in which to invest their time and energy. This book aims to be a guide or roadmap that decodes what it takes to be a CMO.

My second audience is new CMOs who are still growing in their role. They need to know what leadership qualities they must acquire or learn to be effective in their new position. I made more than a few mistakes as a young CMO and now want to help others avoid potential pitfalls, so that they can become highly effective in a short time frame.

My third audience is health care organizations. They need to understand the growing importance of this C-suite position. Did you know that non–health care companies such as Microsoft, Google, and CVS (to name just a few) are hiring CMOs? I can't emphasize enough how underutilized the role has been and how it might be used more extensively and effectively. It's a *rapidly* expanding role!

I have dedicated a significant portion of the book's final chapter to exploring the complexities of leading amidst gender bias. Organizations can take effective steps to support female leadership, steps that do not hinder the individual's growth as a leader. As a female physician leader, I felt it necessary to address this topic in an abbreviated way. I hope to encourage other female physician leaders who may want to pursue the CMO role, as well as give some life-tested counsel to the health care institutions that desire to help such leaders thrive.

Finally, I am indebted to my mentors, each of whom has paved the way for my professional growth. I feel deeply grateful for their significant contributions to my life and career. I have learned a lot from all of them—and now it is my time to pay it forward.

PART 1

The Role of a Chief Medical Officer

The CMO is a pivotal leader who bridges clinical and administrative functions within a health care organization. The position demands influence, relationship-building skills, and the ability to navigate complex interdisciplinary dynamics to promote quality and patient safety. This role has evolved from overseeing credentialing to becoming a strategic partner in health care delivery, quality improvement, and organizational culture.

Part 1 begins by walking us through the evolution of physician leadership, from Victorian times to the current complex health care environment. It then makes a call for physicians to get involved in leadership roles for one simple reason: High-quality and zero-harm patient safety will not be achieved without physician engagement. Additionally, if we want to spur the change that we want to see, we must be at the decision-making table. Someone much wiser than all of us combined, Mahatma Gandhi, said it best: "You must be the change you wish to see in the world."

1

PHYSICIAN LEADERSHIP: A BRIEF HISTORY

Imhotep, who lived around 2600 BCE in ancient Egypt, is often regarded as the first recorded physician. His contributions went beyond medicine, however—he was also a high priest, an architect, and an advisor to Pharaoh Djoser.

Hippocrates is traditionally referred to as "the Father of Medicine." The Hippocratic school revolutionized ancient Greek medicine, establishing it as a discipline distinct from other fields with which it had traditionally been associated (e.g., theurgy and philosophy). He thus established medicine as its own profession.

"Chief medical officer" is the title used in many countries for the senior government official designated as the head of medical services, sometimes at the national level. The position of chief medical officer dates back to Victorian times, although the equivalent title may go by different names across various countries. In the United States, for example, the CMO is called the surgeon general, while in Canada, the CMO is called the chief public health officer. The post is held by a physician who advises and leads a team of medical experts on matters of public health importance.

Physician leadership has undergone a profound transformation over the past few decades. Once confined to clinical excellence and departmental oversight, today's physician leaders are expected to be strategic partners, operational drivers, and cultural stewards. This evolution reflects the growing complexity of health care systems, the demand for integrated care, and the need for leadership that bridges clinical insight with administrative acumen.

This chapter provides a brief historical overview of the evolution of physician leadership roles in the United States, focusing primarily on the role of the CMO. It traces the transformation of physician leadership from early medical practice to the complex administrative and strategic roles seen today.

Early Medical Practice and the Rise of Hospital Medicine

Nicholas Chadi summarized for us the medical situation leading up to the last few decades:

> Merely two hundred years ago, American and European medical treatments were generally provided by independent physicians who went from home to home to offer their services. From this form of medicine, often referred to as "bedside medicine," Western countries started to move towards a more centralized form of medical care provision: hospital medicine.
>
> During the 20th century, as cities steadily grew larger and more populated, numerous hospital super complexes with complicated hierarchal structures emerged. Employing hundreds and sometimes thousands of health care professionals, hospitals became increasingly difficult to manage and required the presence of a well-organized management staff.[1]

A key part of that "well-organized management staff" is the chief medical officer. To help set the stage for the role a CMO plays in the rapidly changing landscape of contemporary health care, let's take a quick tour through the last few decades. We'll soon see that what we know as a CMO today looked *very* different in the not-too-distant past.

The Key Role of Academic Medicine

Long ago, academic medical centers solved the problem of finding and training physicians willing to take on administrative roles beyond their clinical work. This academic model for physicians, according to *Becker's Clinical Leadership*, involves "splitting time between clinical responsibilities and academic responsibilities that include research, teaching, quality improvement, hospital operations and/or strategic planning."[2]

What has evolved over decades into the CMO role, then, began in academic medicine. Physicians were (and still are) taught to master their clinical craft and how to take on additional administrative roles without upending their own work-life balance. "The formula is mutually beneficial," *Becker's* says, "allowing physicians to engage in work that aligns with their specialty and then publish or teach on that subject, which benefits the medical center."[3] Leaders at six academic medical centers contacted by *Becker's* estimated that at least half of their physicians held some type of dual role, whether as clinical leaders, faculty members, department chairs, or physician researchers. *Becker's* explains,

> In some cases, a person might lead a short-term, highly focused project for six months to a year before returning to full-time clinical work. These projects are often entry points into leadership for physicians. . . . Regardless of position, most clinicians in academic centers are dedicated to what's called the triple mission: research, education, and patient care—plus administration . . . this combined mission creates a culture that encourages intertwining work. . . . After decades of managing and creating split roles, academic centers have found several best practices that community hospitals can use.[4]

Paul Wallach, MD, serves as the vice chancellor for health sciences education and the executive vice dean for academic affairs at the University of Pittsburgh School of Medicine. "As an internist," he said, "I had students and residents working alongside me during their clerkships, participating in clinical care. Yes, I gave lectures and led conferences, but it was all integrated. It felt continuous and seamless . . . like anything new, people learn. These are smart, capable physicians and these are learnable skills. They can learn how to incorporate learners onto their teams in ways that are efficient and effective. In fact, residents and students can often help speed up parts of the day. So it's about openness—recognizing that these activities aren't just added tasks, but meaningful work in their own right."[5]

Academic medical centers played a pivotal role in preparing physicians for leadership, and the insights gained are now contributing to advances across the entire health care sector. But what was effective five years ago may not be applicable today (even in academia!), largely because of the changing requirements for this role.

Physician Leadership in the 1990s

Physician leadership has undergone countless changes in just the past few decades. I've seen this transformation firsthand, as have many others. "The American healthcare landscape has undergone a transformational change over the past two decades," said David Nash, MD, MBA, a contributing writer to *MedPage Today*, "and there has been a parallel evolution in the role of the physician executive."[6]

The role of CMO started to become more prevalent in the 1990s—that's when the title was first used—but at that time, it was still considered only a senior medical leader position.[7] The reigning attitude was essentially, "Let the physicians practice medicine and the administrators run the hospital." The CMO served primarily as a liaison between the physician staff and the administration, tasked with translating medical terminology and practices to those who ran the health care facility, along with relaying physician concerns and requests to upper management. According to one organization that offers AI services to hospitals and physicians, doctors historically were seen as solitary figures who focused primarily on patient care in clinical settings.[8]

In a 2024 podcast called *Advancing Health*, hosted by the American Hospital Association (AHA), Dr. Chris DeRienzo, the senior vice president and chief physician executive at the AHA, spoke about the evolving role of physician leaders. DeRienzo spent ten years working as a health system CMO and chief quality officer after working clinically as a neonatologist. He sees essentially three phases of evolution in physician leadership, starting in the 1990s. Consider his description of the first phase (we'll consider the second two phases later in this chapter):

> We've had medical staff privileges and credentials and a medical executive committee for decades. I'm not really talking about the elected leadership role. I'm talking about the earliest members with protected administrative time, who sat on that leadership team. In the eighties and nineties, that . . . typically was an incredibly well-respected physician, had been on staff for maybe twenty or thirty years, was loved by the community and loved by the team. They were given a small office somewhere in the corner and told, "Go listen to the doctors and keep them out of the administration." That was the early phase efforts at engagement. It was a very tightly focused position on medical staff and medical affairs.[9]

Credentialing and Privileging

Another major part of the CMO's job is focused on credentialing and privileging, a critical function that continues to play an equally important role today. While the CMO position has expanded beyond credentials and privilege, this function remains as vital as ever.

From the beginning, CMOs were given the critical job of verifying the credentials of physicians and conveying to them appropriate privileges. Nobody else is in a position to do this well. Poorly done, it can land a hospital in ruinous litigation.

Hospitals have a legal duty to hire only qualified and competent health care providers. Credentialing begins at the Central Verification Office upon the submission of an initial application. The completed file is sent to the medical staff office, and privileges are released after review by the medical staff credentialing committee. It is the CMO's responsibility to oversee and advise the credentialing committee.

Negligent credentialing refers to the failure of a health care organization to properly verify and assess the qualifications of medical staff members. This negligence sometimes occurs when hospitals fail to confirm that a staff member is licensed, competent, and current in their professional training. If that staff member engages in an activity that leads to patient harm, the hospital may be held liable for damages. Hospitals can be found legally negligent if they fail to exercise reasonable care in selecting and evaluating their medical staff.

When an adverse event occurs, investigators will thoroughly examine the credentialing file of the physician involved. Data points, such as a negative reference from a peer or a physician's prior history of adverse outcomes at other institutions, should be thoroughly reviewed and investigated by the credentialing committee.

It's *extraordinarily* important that the credentialing committee, led by the CMO, acts as the hospital's gatekeeper. It's not hard to see why it's remained a traditional role of the CMO ever since the position came into existence.

The first legal case, finding a hospital liable for negligent credentialing occurred in 1965.[10] In *Darling v. Charleston Community Memorial Hospital*, the plaintiff broke his leg during a football game and was treated by an on-call physician, who put the injured man's leg in a cast. The patient subsequently developed gangrene, resulting in the amputation of the leg. The plaintiff sued the hospital for negligence, both because it failed to properly review the physician's work and because a hospital nurse failed to administer some appropriate tests. The court ruled that the hospital failed to act in a reasonably careful manner, which resulted in the patient receiving insufficient care contrary to the hospital's accreditation.

Another major case occurred in 1991 that demonstrated the serious consequences of a physician failing to disclose all relevant information on a job application. In *Johnson v. Misericordia Community Hospital,* the plaintiff had hip surgery in which a physician damaged the man's main femoral nerve and artery, resulting in permanent damage and paralysis to the patient's left leg.[11] The patient first settled the case with his physician and then sued the hospital, claiming it failed to properly verify the physician's credentials.

The physician had wrongly stated in his job application that his privileges had never "been suspended, diminished, revoked, or not renewed" at other hospitals. He also neglected to answer any questions about his malpractice insurance. The hospital had not, in fact, verified the information on the physician's application. If it had, it would have found that the physician's prior hospitals had limited his privileges. Just as bad, if not worse, by failing to verify relevant medical malpractice data, Misericordia hired a physician who already had been subject to *seven* malpractice suits.

Can you see why, although the CMO position has changed greatly since the 1990s, it very much remains the duty of every CMO to carefully oversee a hospital's credentialing and privileging function? This will remain a crucial aspect of the CMO role even as health care continues to rapidly evolve.

I read recently about a huge judgment handed down by an Oklahoma county jury, subsequently affirmed on appeal. The court found a hospital guilty of reckless and intentional negligent credentialing. As a result, it rendered a mammoth judgment of $15 million in compensatory damages, along with $30 million in punitive damages.[12] The physician at the center of the suit had not provided the hospital with proof of current clinical competence to perform a Sistrunk procedure to remove a thyroglossal duct cyst. The four-year-old boy who underwent the procedure subsequently suffered a life-altering injury.

His family alleged that the hospital had allowed an unqualified surgeon to perform the surgery. I offer such details not to heighten the drama of such a tragedy, but to reiterate the crucial role of the CMO in credentialing and privileging.

Since the 1990s, the duties of the CMO have expanded, its scope has grown, and its importance has vastly increased. Nevertheless, credentialing and privileging remain a core, vital function. A patient's safety and a hospital's financial integrity depend on it.

Physician Leadership in the 2000s

In the 2000s, CMOs took on responsibilities for quality and safety alongside credentialing, often collaborating with nursing leaders.

While the CMO title spread in that decade, it tended to be used indiscriminately, referring both to executives focused primarily on brand and communications and to lead physicians beginning to get involved in hospital strategy.[13] David Nash sees this decade as another distinguishable period in the evolution of the CMO:

> In 2000, the typical physician executive was a clinical expert who focused on advancing best clinical practices. Often a renowned research leader in a specialty field, the traditional physician leader was a medical director who served as liaison between the hospital and the credentialed medical staff. Because quality and performance were key aspects of the role, it was important that these leaders be recognized by their peers as high-quality physicians.[14]

Chris DeRienzo saw this decade as phase two in the evolution of the CMO role, "as the ACA passed and the quality movement in health care began to reach a fairly significant crescendo, to where CEOs and boards started saying, 'Okay, doctor, we need you to lead quality as well,' oftentimes in partnership with a chief nurse."[15]

The first dyad roles began to emerge in the 2000s, along with adding more quality and safety and patient-experience work. Still, CMOs were not yet included in most health systems' strategic or operational activities.

The seeds already were sown, however, for additional changes. Writing in 2009, Chadi explained that with the aging of Western populations, "developed countries now [faced] major problems within their healthcare systems," particularly with economics and efficiency. How could they restrain the rising costs of health care coverage? Dramatic changes in a physician's daily routine over a single generation revealed that "the individual orientation that doctors were trained for [did] not fit with the demands of current healthcare systems."[16]

Chadi also suggested that "medical leadership" should have "fully trained physicians occupying leadership roles relevant to the practice of medicine," which he thought might include resource management, decision-making, recruiting, and medical consulting. He also thought these physicians should have a hand in implementing changes and improvements in hospital and clinical settings. He also thought medical leadership should include team-building activities and "an appropriate sharing of decision power."[17]

Chadi quoted Richard Schwartz, a physician with an MBA working for the Kentucky College of Medicine, who declared, "Precisely because they are at the center of clinical service and delivery, physicians are the ideal leaders for healthcare in the 21st century."[18]

Near the end of the decade, Chadi could claim that in "developed countries, very few Chief Executive Officers [were] from a clinical background and even fewer of them [were] medically qualified." So, he suggested that "the CMO can be seen as a facilitator who allows a better interaction between the hospital healthcare professionals and the management team." He then quoted a 2005 article that declared, "The CMO generally has specific duties related to the management, direction, and evaluation of quality initiatives and clinical affairs, but is increasingly involved with the strategic planning and relationship with critical physician groups."[19]

By the end of the 2000s, CMOs began to be recognized as ideal leaders due to their central role in clinical service and delivery. Thus began the metamorphosis of this critical and underutilized role, inching ever closer to what we see today.

Physician Leadership in the 2010s

As the first decade of the twenty-first century wound down, the changing nature of health care made clear the need for physicians at a senior leadership level. CMOs gradually started to become key members of the core administration, providing medical expertise to aid in organizational decisions, especially regarding operational efficiency and strategic alignment. David Nash wrote:

> By 2010, physician executive positions were being filled by "interdisciplinary pioneers" who promoted collaboration and multisectoral research initiatives, and approached health and patient care holistically. As the role became more complex, physician executives were often given the title of vice president of medical affairs.
>
> As the healthcare landscape continued its metamorphosis, so did the role of the physician executive. The job description soon called for a trusted business executive with considerable administrative and financial obligations. By 2018, the position required a strategic partner with a firm understanding of business and healthcare—an MBA degree was a real plus. Candidates were expected to show a track record of innovative and strategic leadership early in their careers (e.g., reimbursement/care models, health policy, community outreach). In addition to being respected by clinicians, the physician executive was expected to represent the views of

all stakeholders and be adept at consensus building, effective communication and negotiation.[20]

Regarding this period, the *Harvard Business Review* declared that CMOs were "expected to creatively apply insights to business challenges, validate decisions with data, create seamless customer experiences across media and revenue channels, and lead efforts to put the customer at the center throughout the organization. Most CMOs [at this time] sit on executive committees and report directly to the CEO. But there is confusion about the role, leading some to question the title and explore alternatives like chief customer officer, chief customer experience officer, and chief growth officer."[21]

Writing in 2018, Martha Sonnenberg, MD, MS, declared that there was "a sea change occurring in American hospitals and health care organizations. We are witnessing a radically changing health care environment in which . . . patients and payers, as well as state and federal governments, are demanding improved quality and safety, and cost containment. In this environment, the traditional hospital organization, as well as organized medical staffs, based as they are in a traditional autonomous role for physicians, are struggling to provide and sustain responsible quality and cost-effective care to patients. . . . It has fallen primarily to the chief medical officer to . . . form a meaningful and operational liaison between hospital administrators and physicians."[22]

Over the previous twenty years, Sonnenberg said the CMO role had "evolved far beyond peer review and privileging, to include utilization review, program growth and development, practice acquisition, integrating health systems, and aligning and coordinating ambulatory inpatient care, technology acquisition and implementation, process improvement, and regulatory compliance."[23] Still, Sonnenberg admitted that during this period, the CMO role was "neither well-defined nor critical." She observed that it was "frequently filled by a senior physician, often as a part-time position, who functioned primarily to influence staff physicians to perform at higher standards and to accept administrative policies." This individual was usually well-liked and respected by peers and therefore trusted to represent medical staff personnel in administrative matters. However, their focus remained "primarily on medical staff issues such as peer review, credentialing and privileging," and they "rarely had strategic or operational responsibility, let alone accountability."[24]

The CMO position became increasingly full-time by 2018. The person in the job had to "demonstrate an ability to deliver with respect to engaging and aligning medical staff, improving performance metrics, improving quality of care and at the same time curtailing costs by more efficient use of resources."[25] By then, CMOs were being encouraged to obtain degrees in business and management or certification from various organizations, such as the American Association for Physician Leadership. Sonnenberg insisted that "above all, the CMO needs a clear understanding of how his or her organization functions . . . and how it may evolve." She recommended that any individual interested in the job should have the ability to assess where and how to break down "clinical or administrative silos" and to determine whether the clinical staff was adequate for successfully achieving such tasks.[26]

"The CMO is, ultimately, like the orchestra conductor," she declared, before concluding:

> Without that role, we may have many expert performers and a beautifully written score, but we do not have the symphonic music that delights the listener. . . . The CMO's role is no longer a luxury, but a necessity for the successful functioning of today's hospitals and health care organizations.[27]

By the end of the 2010s, academia recognized the CMO role as an opportunity. Several institutions began offering dual residency programs that included both a master's in medicine and a master's degree in business. Residents graduating with both an MD/DO and an MBA became ideal candidates for future leadership roles. Thus began the launch of the next generation of physician leaders.

Physician Leadership in the Early 2020s

Since the COVID-19 pandemic (2020–2023), health care systems have recognized the critical importance of physician leadership in all aspects of health care, including in the C-suite. The CMO's role has expanded notably over the past few years and changed significantly in the last decade.

The pandemic heightened the need for physician leadership. And who better to tackle a clinical dilemma than physicians themselves? They took this on as a challenge. Physician leaders were tasked with developing and implementing effective change management strategies. Clinicians developed innovative techniques that had never existed. Scientists found a new way to develop vaccines, and in under a year! This was unheard of.

No doubt you remember what you were doing the day you had your first COVID-positive patient on your campus. I was serving as CMO when our initial patient was admitted on Friday, March 13, 2020, at 4 p.m. We all had goosebumps, and the incident sent shivers down the spines of our clinicians. We thought we were prepared . . . but just like other institutions, we had to modify systems and pivot quickly to meet the demands of evolving science. ER physicians manned the front lines, wearing full personal protective equipment. Anesthesiologists wore N95s, and intensivists intubated critically ill patients at their own risk.

This challenge took a huge toll on the physician community. While it brought us together, it did so at an enormous cost. I remember reading about a young ED physician who committed suicide, as she could not handle the pressures of the pandemic. Taking care of sick individuals and seeing so much death is a heavy burden—and this is where the role of the CMO became critical.

How do we provide support to our teams in the trenches? Such support could mean equipment, peer support, counseling, and certainly keeping everyone updated on the new remedies constantly being released. I have no doubt that in those years, the realization came home to hospitals across the world: CMOs are essential players in the administration of health care organizations, contributing enormously to operational efficiency and patient-centered care.

Since then, chief medical officers have taken on executive leadership roles and continue to gain opportunities for further development. CMOs are key to the success of any health care organization, serving as an indispensable link between clinical and nonclinical departments. And yet, the position's primary responsibility has not changed: The CMO remains the loudest voice for quality and patient safety in any room.

I have served in the CMO role for more than seven years. When I began, the expectation was little more than, "Just do peer review and credentials and stay in your lane of physicianship." How times have changed! And I am ecstatic about that. I understand what David Nash means when he says:

> By the time 2020 rolled around, innovation was name of the game. In addition to research and clinical excellence, a physician executive had to demonstrate the ability to apply that expertise and expand thought leadership into patient/consumer experience, primary healthcare, digital health, and technology transfer/venture initiatives. The job had become onerous for even the most talented and energetic among us!
>
> We all know what came next—the unprecedented upheaval and irreversible changes that came about as a result of the pandemic. The post-pandemic health care delivery system will continue to evolve rapidly. What are the implications for "who's at the helm"?[28]

My Personal Journey in Physician Leadership

To help you better understand my perspective in this book, allow me to give you a glimpse into my personal journey. From a girl in a small town in northern India to a practicing female physician in the United States, I now serve as a CMO in an exceptional health care system.

I came to the US in 2000, which means I've spent half my life in India and the other half in America. I finished medical school and an internal medicine residency in India. While serving as chief resident in New Delhi, I decided to pursue further opportunities in health care by taking the USMLE examination and subsequently received a pre-match offer from a program in Illinois. I worked in an underserved area for seven years on a J-1 visa. During this period, I expanded my skills beyond clinical medicine. Working with the chief operating officer, I presented my first business plan. I got certified in utilization medicine, was elected as the medical staff treasurer, and gained experience in governance. I worked first in primary care and later as the hospitalist medical director.

After seven years, I transitioned to academic medicine and became an associate program director of an internal medicine residency program, which gave me exposure to graduate medical education (GME) governance (and its challenges). At that time, I had to choose whether to pursue academics or further my career in a non-GME route. I chose the latter and enrolled in an MBA program. Four and a half years later, I obtained my certification.

Since my move to the States, I've remained in the Midwest, first in Illinois and now in Kansas. While I've always enjoyed practicing bedside medicine, after more than twenty years of clinical practice under my belt, I decided to explore other avenues so I could impact health care on a larger scale. That, truly, was my motivation for even *thinking* about becoming a CMO. I saw that influencing quality and tackling clinicians' daily challenges required me to be involved in decision-making.

To guide my thinking, I started getting involved in various committees at the hospital, where I quickly learned that there is *so* much more than bedside medicine! Through my committee work, I gained exposure to fields not covered during residency. Participating in care management and on the utilization management committee helped me realize that physicians must become better stewards, not only regarding the health of their patients, but also as financial stewards of health care itself. Physicians have an *enormous* impact, not only in their small sphere but also on global health care. Modern medicine is very expensive, and sometimes we physicians contribute toward that cost, whether intentionally or not. Utilization management revealed how physicians interact with insurance companies and how the added administrative burden can contribute to the hospital's and physicians' financial burnout.

In time, I got board-certified in quality and care management and obtained a green belt in Lean Six Sigma. I needed to learn the tools of process improvement to lead a root cause analysis (RCA) and impact quality in a more meaningful way. I attended leadership courses and invested in my own growth. My employing organization saw my potential and reciprocated by investing in me with additional learning opportunities. I am now and always will be in a lifelong learning environment! That provides the foundation for both clinical and administrative roles.

For seven years, I served as the CMO of two hospitals. Now, I am a regional CMO over four hospitals. It certainly has been a journey! I have learned so much—and yet my journey in leadership has only just begun. I am constantly learning new skill sets with every interaction I have. Six months ago, I wasn't the leader I am now. I'm learning that the evolution of self is critical and translates to an enhanced leadership style.

I didn't get here on my own, of course. I have relied on many peers for guidance and have been fortunate to have excellent mentors along the way who have shared pearls of wisdom from their own experiences.

I can't thank them enough! In this book, I'm passing on their knowledge—and mine—for the next generation.

A Long Way Past Ill-Defined

At the very beginning, the idea of physician leadership was extremely ill-defined. Back then, physicians could tap into it only informally and make decisions based on enlightened guesswork.

It's taken us decades to adequately define physician leadership as it relates to the broad field of health care. Today, we have clearly outlined positions, including those with no titles, medical directorships, chief quality officers, CMOs, chief clinical officers, and CEOs.

Physician leaders exist both at the federal government and state levels. Nearly every state in the union has a CMO. Physician leadership is vital to the existence of the Centers for Medicare and Medicaid Services, the National Institutes of Health (NIH), and the Agency for Healthcare Research and Quality (AHRQ), to name a few. Every insurance company has a market CMO, and every large tech corporation has a CMO who leads the conversation in emerging technologies, including artificial intelligence. Throughout health care in this country, we now have clearly defined physician leadership roles.

My question for you is this: Where do you think you may best fit in the broad landscape of contemporary physician leadership? And where would you *like* to fit?

2

THE EXPANDING ROLE OF THE CMO

It's hard to believe how few chief medical officer positions existed until just a few years ago. Online recruiting company Zippia claims that 9,520 individuals were employed as CMOs in 2016. That number rose to 12,519 by 2025.[29] Zippia predicts CMO roles will grow by 28 percent from 2018 to 2028, adding about 136,200 new jobs over ten years.[30]

Back in September 2022, the American Association for Physician Leadership noted, "Shortly after passage and implementation of the Affordable Care Act [in 2010], AAPL recognized a rapid increase in organizations seeking to employ physicians and educate physician leaders. The trend has continued."[31] I agree with the AAPL when it says:

> Healthcare evolution requires physicians with leadership experience to guide change. A career in medical leadership has become a positive choice for female as well as male physicians. In addition to having excellent physicians at the core of the healthcare system clinically, a compelling case can be made for a physician leader who possesses the skills and knowledge about the organization of medical care and can act as liaison among all those with an interest in medicine, including patients, healthcare providers, insurers, economists, and other administrators.[32]

The *Journal of the American Medical Association* said in 2022 that it was "seeing a trend of corporations implementing" the CMO position, including huge businesses such as Google, Tyson Foods, Delta, Royal Caribbean, BP, Woolworths, Uber, and even the National Football League. It added that the popular press had reported "an almost 19% increase in CMO postings in recent years as companies of all types [considered] implementing the role."[33]

Perhaps it is no surprise, then, that executive recruiting firm Russell Reynolds declares, "As the healthcare industry rapidly evolves and top medical talent becomes scarce, the MedTech industry is facing a shortage of experienced chief medical officer (CMO) successors. To successfully meet the clinical and business demands of this complex role, CEOs and current CMOs must begin proactively preparing the next generation of medical leaders."[34] The firm then added, "While there is no single set of competencies that guarantee success in the CMO position, we found that organizations consistently seek leaders with clinical expertise, the ability to foster effective collaboration across functions, strong business acumen, enterprise-level thinking, effective executive communication skills, and digital literacy when looking for their next CMO."[35]

What does it mean to succeed as a chief medical officer in the second quarter of the twenty-first century? In this chapter, we'll review each of the elements just named, along with others. The CMO position has significantly changed in recent years and will continue to evolve to meet the needs of the health care system. As value-based payment models become more prevalent—and, might I say, could replace fee-for-service completely—CMOs are poised to lead and impact this dramatic change. I'd like to highlight several relatively new (and yet key) characteristics of the current job:

- a strong focus on quality,
- a need to collaborate on strategy,
- an acceptance of the C-suite role, and
- a push for new education and training.

Let's explore each of these facets in greater detail.

A Strong Focus on Quality

Since the COVID-19 pandemic, it has become clear how much we need physicians in expanded leadership roles. The CMO position has rapidly evolved from focusing on credentialing and privileges to becoming the key voice in leading quality.

During the pandemic, I was able to show our own C-suite how the chief nursing officer and I, working hand in hand, demonstrated the critical significance of clinical dyad leadership, where physician and nursing leaders collaborate to enhance quality. None of us works on an island! While it is true historically that quality and safety have been viewed as vaguely important, physicians today play a crucial role in these areas. They simply *must* be engaged—and the CMO, as the physician leader, must lead this process.

In his 2019 book *Five Disciplines for Zero Patient Harm*, author Charles A. Mowll, who worked for more than twenty years as an executive VP at the Joint Commission, criticized the US health care system for its long failure to articulate a vision and strategic plan for how the system should work, and for neglecting to lay out its quality and cost-control objectives. This had begun to change with the 2010 enactment of the Affordable Care Act, which required the secretary of the US Department of Health and Human Services to establish the nation's first health care quality improvement plan, eventually called the National Strategy for Quality Improvement in Health Care (the National Quality Strategy, for short). The first National Quality Strategy was issued in March 2011 as one of three broad national aims to "improve the overall quality, by making health care more patient-centered, reliable, accessible, and safe."[36] Citing the unacceptably high numbers of health care–associated infections (1.7 million), resulting deaths (99,000), and adverse medication-related events (770,000) each year, the National Quality Strategy stated that "health care–related errors harm millions of American patients each year and needlessly add billions of dollars to health care costs." The first strategy was called the Making Care Safer initiative, which formally established the national goal of zero patient harm:

> Health care providers should be relentless in their efforts to reduce the risk for injury from care, aiming for zero harm whenever possible and striving to create a system that reliably provides high-quality health care for everyone.[37]

And who better to lead and positively impact the "zero preventable harm" journey than the chief medical officer of an organization?

As I've stated, when I first accepted the role of CMO several years ago, the expectation from my own C-suite was merely to "oversee credentials and privileging." But very quickly, executive partners realized the underutilization of my role. My colleagues and I established a safety event review system, developed a peer review process, standardized procedures for debriefing health care infections, and implemented quality improvement plans. I also created a quality and patient safety curriculum for the residency programs on our campus. Training focused on quality and zero harm, which ideally should begin early in a medical professional's education (this final point could fill an entire book by itself).

Remember, the CMO is the *loudest* clinical voice in the administrative corridor! It's an extremely important voice because we so easily forget that clinical quality is a hospital's *only* product. Every company, including health care organizations, needs to deliver quality products if it hopes to compete for market share. *Everything* follows quality.

This position has grown significantly in recent years. The chief medical officer is now regarded as the leading authority on quality and patient safety, with responsibilities that extend across nearly every department within the hospital. And yet, the role continues to be underutilized, either because top executives still haven't seen its true utility or because CMOs themselves have yet to appreciate the full value and potential of their position. The latter is an intriguing statement, and this book aims to offer clarity for current and future CMOs.

CMOs use various approaches to fulfill their responsibilities. The two following examples demonstrate this reality and show how these differences affect the processes for disclosing information and addressing patient concerns.

One director of risk mentioned that her region had more than one CMO. A situation arose in which a grieving family sent a letter to the CMO of the hospital where a patient had died. The director of risk's department knew about the letter because they had already responded to the family. The situation involved a very sick patient with a complex medical history who was actively dying. Since such a situation is difficult to explain in a letter, the director of risk asked the CMO, "As the chief medical officer, could you please call this family's daughter and talk to her, in hopes of giving her closure?"

"No," the CMO replied. "I don't know anything about this case. I was not involved in it. What would I have to say? It should come from the providers involved in the case."

The problem was that the daughter had grown very angry with those providers, which meant that such a conversation would not likely be beneficial.

"I was extremely disappointed that the CMO did not want to get involved to help us with this scenario," said the director of risk. "We sent another resolution letter, but I would have liked it to have been a phone call from the CMO."

Fortunately, the same director of risk had a positive example to share. In a similar scenario, the hospital sent a letter to a family who felt upset with the provided care. She approached the second CMO and asked, "Can you help us out here? This one doctor is not good at communicating with patients and families. That would not be a helpful phone call."

"No problem," the CMO answered. "I will connect with the medical director of the ICU as well."

The medical director of the ICU called, as did that CMO. The hospital wrote a follow-up letter to the family, the second CMO reviewed it and made edits, and the letter was sent off.

"That's the kind of thing I need," the director of risk said.[38]

The differing approaches in similar cases by the two CMOs affected both patient issue resolution and collaboration with the director of risk management. It would be valuable to examine the perspectives of both chief medical officers; the individual with a deeper comprehension of the role appeared to generate a notably more positive impact.

Employed vs. Contracted Physician Groups

You cannot discuss the quality of care without taking into consideration the team members in the trenches who deliver that care. Although a CMO oversees a hospital's physician workforce, "oversees" takes on a different meaning depending on whether the physicians are employed or contracted.

In academic hospitals, most medical staff are directly employed by the institution. Examples include the Mayo Clinic, Cleveland Hospital, Johns Hopkins, and other university hospitals. It's the reverse in community settings, with the majority of physicians being independent. Independents are classified as contracted, aligned with a clinically integrated network, or unaligned. Physician groups commonly contracted to provide coverage for multiple departments include emergency medicine, pathology, and radiology, among others. There are also independent physician groups on the medical staff who are not part of a clinically integrated network. They manage their own patients and are less aligned.

The medical staff is a completely different entity from nurses or other employees who are governed by the hospital's policies. The medical staff is an independent body with its own bylaws, rules, and regulations, each with their own variables. The complexity of aligning such a diverse group is no easy task! It requires special skills and a unique mindset.

Keep this in mind as you think about becoming a CMO. In most hospital settings, you will have to manage and direct your colleagues through *influence* and not *control.*

This explains why relationships matter so much in the CMO position. The biggest body that the CMO oversees is the medical staff, which (as a whole) doesn't report to the CMO. Although you will directly manage hospital departments such as quality, risk, care management, or clinical documentation—all of which play a role in enhancing care delivery—it is the physicians in the trenches who have the greatest impact on quality. And the *only* way to influence change is by building trust and relationships. This is a learned skill at the core of every successful CMO. You must learn to use your *influence* to change behavior.

Jason Golbin, DO, executive vice president and CMO of Long Island, New York–based Catholic Health, states that "the never-ending focus is on quality, patient safety and the principles of high reliability. Most every discussion I engage in is grounded in clinical compassion and empathy for the patient, and thus focused on driving quality, safety and the patient experience. That's the CMO's most strategic endeavor."[39] Golbin sees the CMO role as "deeply rooted in clinical leadership. [CMOs] are responsible for ensuring that the care delivered across the entire health system is safe, patient-centered, high-quality, evidence-based, and at the same time fully aligned with strategic goals."[40]

Medical Executive Leadership

Achieving this goal requires active participation from medical staff and physician leaders, which is the key to success for all CMOs in any organization. I have been privileged to work with smart, intelligent medical staff presidents and others. It is crucial to have a good working relationship with the medical executive team, which in all hospitals traditionally includes the department chairs and other ad hoc leaders.

One important function of a CMO is to educate, guide, and engage with the medical executive committee. Without them on your side, you will fail. The only way to get them engaged is by being transparent and closing the loop in a timely manner. Doing this will quickly gain their trust. But medical executives can be daunting to lead or guide! They openly express their thoughts and grievances. I can safely say from my own experience (by being on both sides of the coin) that the only time physicians "lose their cool" is when patient care is negatively impacted. If we as CMOs can show progress or explain the "why" for a decision that they disagree with, they will still respect us for being honest with them. Physicians are among the smartest of human beings, and they appreciate our honesty as a show of respect toward them and their intellect.

A Need to Collaborate on Strategy

CMOs across health care are becoming part of strategy, and rightfully so. Who is better qualified to decide which clinical services are safe on campus?

The CMO assembles clinical and nonclinical teams for failure mode and effects analysis (FMEA) to ensure a safe approach before launching new services. This is a critical and (unfortunately) often forgotten tool in the armamentarium of any patient safety leader—and no one is better positioned to lead the FMEA before the start of new services than the chief medical officer.

You simply can't go in cold and say, "We're going to do brain surgery today." You must instead first ask, "Do we have the components to do brain surgery? Do we have the required nursing competencies? Do we have the necessary equipment? Do we have the essential OR structure? Do we have an adequate programmatic strategy behind the services, or do we need to build one?" That's all *strategy*, and that's where CMOs are getting involved.

Allen Verrill, an MD and a hospital system CEO, believes that all CMO candidates must grasp that they are part of the executive team. As such, they *will* be involved with strategy. They are not there merely to inform administrators about how doctors do things. CMOs are "increasingly central to a broad range of financial and strategic decisions, requiring them to make recommendations regarding evolving aspects of health care delivery," declared a 2022 *JAMA Health Forum* article.[41]

Let me give you an example. In a previous hospital, our executive team wanted to build a neuroendovascular service line, which required collaboration across departments. The approach that we took was to evaluate for people, plant, and equipment (PP&E). As a CMO, I partnered with all disciplines, including the COO, the service line, and department leaders. We brought everyone into one room and explored various scenarios, from admission to discharge. We discussed equipment, nursing staff, technologist competencies, clinical protocols, and the availability of a board-certified physician.

CMOs play a significant role in such strategic discussions. We must be willing to say, "Nope, we don't have a board-certified physician with the right fellowship. We'd have to get one," and "Nope, we don't have a biplane CT where the procedure can be performed safely."

In our case, we connected the intensivists and the proceduralists in one room to review pre- and post-op order sets for such complex cases. We identified gaps within the EMR that had to be addressed before we started the service line.

I encourage all clinical leaders to regularly use this valuable exercise. If we do this right on the front end, we will have fewer patient errors requiring an RCA on the back end.

As a first step in this process, CMOs typically collaborate with a strategy team to assess community needs. Once those are determined, we then look to find the right physician who can help lead the project. As the CMO, you must remember that you're not "the expert." Rather, you're forming a team you can rely on throughout the process. Deference to expertise is a fundamental principle of high reliability organizations (see chapter 9).

Although the process may sound straightforward, it is anything but, especially for physicians-turned-CMOs who are used to making decisions on their own. Working and leading alone always used to sit at the top of the hierarchical pyramid; now we must learn to build a team and lead with influence. It is tough, but it gets easier as we grow in our leadership journey.

The rapid increase in physician leadership roles across health care organizations has tended to create uncomfortable discussions in leadership circles where leaders traditionally have been nonclinical. Why are these discussions so uncomfortable? Nonclinical administrative leaders are trained in traditional leadership methods. They are taught to be servant leaders, good listeners, and consensus builders. Their administrative training looks *very* different from a medical resident's, whose training demands quick decision-making, is competitive by nature, and expects physicians to have quick answers to all clinical dilemmas. Many traditional leaders are not used to the direct, impatient style that a physician often brings to most discussions. This tends to make some leaders uncomfortable, maybe at times more so if the physician leader happens to be a strong female. I address this issue further in the book, where I dedicate a segment to the topic and speak directly to female physician leaders (see chapter 9).

So, should leadership in medicine undergo a paradigm shift? Are empathy and consensus essential in modern leadership? Or should the soft skills of emotional intelligence take a back seat? Fortunately, this is not a "one or the other" choice. Health care needs *both* kinds of leadership skills in place to navigate the roiling waters ahead. Both quick decision-making *and* traditional soft skills (see chapter 7) will continue to play key roles in impacting the culture of any health care institution, which in turn impacts patient safety and quality.

Physician and former hospital CMO Chris DeRienzo, quoted earlier, says, "By and large, the shift has been to having physician leaders who are true, core partners, not only to the chief nurse, but to the COO, the chief strategy officer, and the CFO, *especially* when it comes to strategy and operations. That's not because the physicians themselves have changed, but because our environment has changed.

The most forward-thinking and/or integrated systems have needed to bring the chief physician into the fold on making the key strategic and operational decisions of the organization."[42]

Because of this new mix of physician and traditional leadership personalities in health care, DeRienzo believes that "on the physician side, the kind of person who we might have appointed to a VP admiral in the nineties or lifted into a chief of quality in the early 2000s might not be the same kind of person who now is willing to engage in the kind of strategy and operational learning that we need to do in order to be fundamental partners at that kind of a table."[43]

Jason Golbin probably encapsulates as well as anyone the idea of CMO-as-strategist when he says, "The role of the chief medical officer has evolved beyond tactical problem-solving to taking on greater responsibility for strategic leadership. The CMO . . . is an integral member of corporate leadership . . . the CMO needs to ensure a winning balance of clinical excellence, operational efficiency and strategic alignment."[44]

A Full Acceptance of the C-Suite Role

In former days, CMOs were not considered (and did not act as) full-fledged members of a health care organization's executive team. Those days have passed. Dr. Allen Verrill says firmly to CMO candidates, "Get serious about becoming a full member of the executive team. You need a basic level of competency in all the different skill sets, just like you expect of others on the team. You are not special as a physician on that team. You're special because you are a necessary member of the team." He adds:

> A lot of times, we have a CFO who runs operations and all the clinical work. We have a COO who runs some clinical operations and does everything else. Somehow, we leave the CMO sitting out, feeling like they can just be the physician in the group. I think that's an injustice to the team.

> In fact, the CMO needs to be as competent in the other core aspects of the senior leadership team as they expect those team members to be in *their* world. It doesn't help the organization if they're not that. This means they may have some humility and curiosity work to do! You don't know as much in these spaces as you think you do; you really don't! I don't know anybody who does until they actually dive into the other person's shoes.[45]

Allen would no doubt receive a loud "Amen!" for expressing such thoughts from Ken Lukhard, a highly successful retired hospital CEO. Ken insisted, "A CMO must be a critical member of the C-suite, involved in all the critical discussions and decisions of the organization. He or she must be viewed by the organization as a critical member of the C-suite, as important as the CFO and the COO and those kinds of positions. The chief medical officer's role must be high-profile and integral to all the operations of the hospital, just like the other members of the C-suite. They all have their areas of expertise, they all have their wheelhouse, but they need to be part of a very collaborative, high-functioning team. That's a must."[46]

The director of risk quoted earlier was not in the room when Allen and Ken gave their take on this issue, but she might as well have been. Listen to her perspective:

> It's important that they understand that being a chief medical officer is not just about the title. They're an administrator, and there are going to be times when they must have crucial conversations with their providers, whether it's about their performance, their behavior, or something related to complaints and grievances filed by patients and their families. Sometimes, they must take an unpopular stance to highlight these perspectives to the provider.

> I have seen many CMOs during my career, and the strongest are about doing what's right, especially regarding patient safety and patient care. *And* they have tough skin.

All this accords with an article in the *Journal of the American Medical Association* that stated physician leaders must "gain experience with the daily operations, norms, expectations, and culture of a corporate environment." These individuals require "knowledge of the company's other functions and operations, relevant policies and standards, and the necessary terminology and facility for collaborating with other corporate leaders (e.g., executives focused on sales, marketing, operations, and finance)."[47] The article asserts that CMOs often feel challenged about "how to successfully integrate health considerations into more traditional business operations, which requires more prolonged, multidimensional exposure to business than typically received in shorter-form trainings."[48]

And where can CMOs get such "prolonged, multidimensional exposure to business"? Currently, this occurs primarily through collaboration, shared learning, and interactions with other C-suite members.

Listen to Dr. Verrill again: "The ideal candidate understands that if they're becoming a CMO, they're becoming a professional executive leader. They're not a physician with leadership skills who is going to help guide the administration to be the translator or ambassador between the medical staff and the administration. That was the old, traditional way CMOs functioned, but I think that's insufficient for today's CMO. They are an executive leader in a hospital's executive C-suite."

To end this section, I'd like you to hear from one more physician-turned-CMO who took on multiple leadership roles at various levels throughout his career, whether in hospitals, at a company, or at the state level. He is a mentor of mine with a remarkably similar perspective to those you've just read. Dr. Rick Scott said:

> Although it's only recently that the CMO was embraced in the C-suite, their perspective crosses the skill sets and backgrounds of the suite's other members in a most unique way. . . . Many physician executives have also been small business owners, built medical groups, contracted with insurers, and learned a good bit about HR issues, marketing, and finance.
>
> The core business of hospitals is to provide high-quality, efficient care in a safe environment to each and every patient. It's what CMOs learned to do in their practice and what made them successful relative to their peers. The need for patient trust and satisfaction is ingrained in the physician member of a C-suite because that's who they are.
>
> And unlike the CEO, CFO, SVP of marketing, and COO, only the physician member of the team knows what it's like to take a trauma patient from the ER through surgery and recovery, a first-time mom through pregnancy to delivery, or the just-diagnosed cancer patient through their choices on a long and frightening journey. No other member of that team has had to break the news to a child's parents that the child's disease would not likely allow them to ever see college, or has had to tell a son that his mom did not make it.
>
> As physicians, we have a deep appreciation not only for how the patient needs to be approached, but for how the family needs care as well. We often know better what marketing may resonate and what may fall flat. And in interactions with the family, we may be the only executive who gets to start from a well-earned position of trust.[49]

And now it's my turn to say, "Amen."

A Push for New Education and Training

Not all physicians make good leaders, at least in part because their schooling taught them that they were the captain of the ship, the general of the army, the king of the empire. They learned a common philosophy: "You do what I say and don't question me."

Given the new realities of health care, is it any wonder that the *Journal of the American Medical Association* has said that "medical training must be reconsidered to ensure physicians are leaders in producing health across a range of career paths"? And how can we best prepare physicians to contribute in a new and more effective way? *JAMA* answers that this "requires reimagining medical training, shifting away from the linear development of increasingly specialized clinical competencies to a broader outcome-focused approach that recognizes and incorporates the many inputs to individual and community health." It admits that "most medical school and residency curricula feature relatively little in the way of training in public health and policy or in the core business and management skills that might be expected of a senior corporate leader." And it concludes that health care "will need to consider new educational programs and training opportunities that can provide individuals the blend of clinical expertise and business acumen needed to succeed in these positions."[50]

Where can the physician leaders of tomorrow acquire such a "blend of clinical expertise and business acumen"? They might begin by looking into one or more already well-established leadership training programs for physicians, including resources from the American Association for Physician Leadership, the Center for Physician Leadership Excellence, and the Healthcare Leadership Institute.

But why not offer such training to students while they are still in medical school? A 2014 survey of medical students in the UK reported that 85 percent of those surveyed thought they should be taught leadership, communication, teamwork, and quality improvement skills in medical school.[51] So, why don't we begin leadership training early in a student's medical education? Why not teach them the fundamentals of various approaches to leadership, including transformational leadership, situational leadership, and servant leadership? I believe the Association of American Medical Colleges gets it right: "Leadership development has never been more essential for navigating and solving the complex challenges facing today's medical schools and academic health systems."[52]

We need physician leaders with both medical expertise *and* excellent management skills, individuals who know how to communicate effectively *and* who have been trained to think both critically and cooperatively in teams. I believe our medical students need to learn, while in school, how nonphysicians think.

Chris DeRienzo would caution both young physicians and medical students, "Do not make the mistake that I've seen many physicians make. They assume that because they become an expert in their pyramid of pediatric endocrinology or interventional cardiology, that makes them an expert in all of health care. There are *so* many things we can still learn and *so* many people willing to teach us, that all it really takes is being open to acknowledging that I don't know a darn thing about supply chain management."[53] DeRienzo also suggests that both students and young physicians learn to say, "I am here to learn, and I want to be a partner and help." DeRienzo said he's watched "door after door after door open for physicians who are willing to take that step" and urges them to adopt an attitude of, "Hey, I know my stuff really, really well—but tell me about yours. Let me learn from you."[54]

Research shows that leadership training is most impactful when integrated early into a student's medical education. AAMC has established leadership development programs for medical students, with two-and-a-half-day seminars that focus on skills such as self-awareness, team communication, and time management. All of these are critically needed once students enter the real world of medicine.[55]

The American Medical Association acknowledges leadership as essential for future physicians and has developed Leadership 101 training modules for medical students.[56] One AMA newswire suggested that medical students will shape the future of this nation's health care delivery, but that while learning the clinical aspects of care is significant, leadership skills are also key to the students' development. I wholeheartedly agree with that statement.

A Considerable Opportunity

I applaud the *Journal of the American Medical Association* for saying, "A broadly oriented CMO role represents a significant departure from the typical physician career path, but one with considerable opportunity to improve the health and well-being of large numbers of people through strategy and operational decisions that influence entire organizations and their stakeholders."[57]

More opportunities exist for today's CMOs to radically improve health care than ever before. We've come a long way in a few short decades, but the future holds possibilities that boggle the mind. If you're serious about pursuing a path to a CMO role, or even if you're just thinking about it, I urge you to listen closely to the words of Dr. David Nash:

> The post-pandemic era will require a new type of physician leader, one who can refocus our attention on performance improvement and inspire the sweeping organizational changes. Yes, we need innovative leaders with additional skill sets including expertise in digital health, technology transfer, and a deeper understanding of the role of private equity in healthcare.
>
> But we also need leaders who are sensitive to diversity, inclusion and, most importantly, reducing disparities and inequities in care. There couldn't be a better time to seek physician

> executives from different backgrounds, cultures, and other demographics.[58]

As a female physician from India now working as a regional CMO in the United States, I must tell you that I could not have said it better myself.

3

YOUNG CMOS HELP DETERMINE HEALTH CARE'S FUTURE

This portion of the book has a very narrow focus. This message is intended for early-career physicians evaluating their professional trajectories and contemplating the possibility of transitioning into health care administration, with a particular focus on the role of chief medical officer. If this describes you, then this chapter is for you, because I want to encourage you to pursue that path.

The big, bold truth is that we need a small army of talented, enthusiastic, thoughtful young physicians who want to help shape the future of health care, not only in the United States but around the world. And it's easy to see why.

The experience and delivery of excellent medicine is changing at lightning speed all over the globe. More than ever, we desperately require younger physicians who excel at their clinical work, who have a deep understanding and appreciation for the business and operational side of health care, *and* who have a passion for fulfilling the promise that modern medicine offers.

We won't get there without you.

Physician Leadership Is Essential

I'm not the only one saying such things, of course. For the last several years, many articles, white papers, highly respected organizations, and accomplished medical personnel have trumpeted the need for legions of younger physicians to bring their expertise, experience, and passion to the administrative corridor. The future of health care depends on it.

A 2022 white paper proclaimed that physician leadership is "more valuable than ever" and declared, "Physician leadership has only become more essential for health care's continued journey toward higher quality, consistent safety, streamlined efficiency and for completing the transformation to value-based medicine."[59]

Rick Guarino, MD, formerly the VP of medical affairs at Wilson Medical Center in Wilson, North Carolina, claimed that physician leadership gives organizations "a competitive differential" and a "definite edge over a hospital that does not have it."[60]

The American Association of Physician Leadership has seen a "strong connection between high-quality ratings and physician leadership" and insists that "an overwhelming number of top-ranked hospitals continue to be run by physician CEOs."[61] It also champions the view that physicians are best suited to lead clinical efforts to achieve true patient-centered care and says that it is well recognized that our society thinks of all physicians as leaders, at least at some level.[62] The organization also includes physician leadership as one of its "nine essential elements required to provide optimal patient-centered care."[63]

Research conducted by Amanda Goodall, PhD, of the University of London, has consistently found that "the best-performing hospitals are led disproportionately by physicians" and that overall hospital quality scores are 25 percent higher when doctors run hospitals.[64]

A study by McKinsey & Company that investigated several factors associated with health care productivity found "an association between higher organizational scores on several management dimensions, with reduced rates of hospital-acquired infection and hospital readmission, greater patient satisfaction, and improved financial margins. The study revealed stronger physician leadership to be a key contributor to this organizational performance: "The hospitals with greater degrees of physician leadership involvement scored higher, on average, in performance management and Lean management, and produced high average overall management scores."[65]

Grace Terrell, MD, the author of the 2022 book *Reframing Contemporary Physician Leadership*, said, "If you look at the top ten health systems in the U.S. as rated by *U.S. News and World Report*, they're almost all physician-led. The vast majority of the systems that are well run have significant physician leadership at the top. Physicians who are able to broaden their point of view beyond the exam room, or the operating room, can become an important driver to push the organizations to where we really need to go as a healthcare delivery system."[66]

Finally, Ken Lukhard, the former CEO of a major health care organization quoted earlier, told me, "It is not possible to achieve a world-class organization, or to benchmark against top performers, without outstanding physician leadership. It really all starts with a great CMO. To me, they're worth every dollar they earn. They're vital to a vibrant, healthy hospital. They just *have* to be in place."

Let's Ignite the Spark of Leadership

Both great challenges and vast opportunities face us in contemporary physician leadership. And one thing is certain: Health care organizations and physicians *must* collaborate to make leadership roles both appealing and effective. Why? For one reason, many observers believe that the number of younger physicians seeking leadership roles is declining. "Physicians' presence in leadership roles within hospitals, health systems and private practice has declined in recent years," declared a 2025 *Becker's Physician Leadership* article, "as increased administrative burdens, burnout and other job pressures make it more difficult for physicians to expand beyond purely clinical responsibilities."[67]

Many contemporary health care leaders have noted that younger physicians seem to be showing less interest today in responsibilities outside of clinical care. While physicians traditionally have balanced full-time clinical loads with extra leadership responsibilities, a greater focus today on work-life balance appears to have made younger physicians more reluctant to take on extra duties. "There's a separation now between their passion for health care and their desire for work-life balance," said Nariman Heshmati, MD, the chief physician and operations executive at Lee Physician Group in Fort Myers, Florida.[68]

Becker's Hospital Review noticed a similar trend at a Pennsylvania health care group, "where younger physicians are striving to achieve work-life balance. However, in achieving that balance, many become less interested in leadership, since it 'seems more like administration, and most younger physicians are uninterested,'" said Sean Reinhardt, MD, the health care group's vice president and chief medical officer.[69]

I believe it's crucial for our younger physicians to understand the administrative or leadership role *in its entirety*. They may perceive the role as consisting primarily of administrative tasks and meetings, rather than recognizing the large and growing opportunities to shape an organization's strategic direction, develop a corporate vision, or lead initiatives designed to enhance quality. I hope to provide some clarity at this point that might help ignite the spark we are all looking for.

Leo Spector, an MD and the CEO of OrthoCarolina in Charlotte, North Carolina, said, "We should see more physicians who are involved with hospital administration or healthcare insurance companies, because at the end of the day, we're the ones caring for the patients. We need to have a strong voice in leadership."[70]

It is well established that physician leadership is essential for any health care company in this era that wants to deliver high-quality, safe care. Health care organizations must make leadership roles more appealing to future generations—but at the same time, physicians must be *open* to taking on these positions before *choosing* them. One without the other will not work.

Allow me to outline a few simple steps designed to address our contemporary need for more physician leadership:

Organizational Initiatives

1. *Invest financially in physician leadership.* Offer stipends and training reimbursement to help young physician leaders acquire essential skills for success.
2. *Emphasize mentorship and make it widely available.* Encourage younger physicians to partner with a senior physician who is invested in the organization and has been in a position of leadership. Encourage the mentors to share their stories and the satisfaction they derived from their actions that positively impacted patient care. Nothing excites physicians more.
3. *Show value in your group's leadership roles and recognize them publicly.* Physicians appreciate recognition, just like anyone else. Motivate them to keep going.
4. *Make it personal.* Share the bigger picture so that they can understand their impact on a broader community beyond their own patient population. Help them understand the bigger "why."
5. *Keep them engaged in decision-making projects.* This is the biggest motivator for all clinicians, and it is the quickest way to get their buy-in. Involving physicians in the design of a project shows them respect and transparency.

Physician Initiatives

1. *Invest both time and resources in building young physician leaders.* Some of the onus here is on the physicians themselves; you must fully engage to better grasp the role.
2. *Encourage self-investment.* Physicians need to learn the business aspect of medicine. Earn a master's degree (or an advanced

degree in an area essential to health care) in addition to your MD or DO. This should be a physician/hospital partnership and a shared financial investment.

3. *Focus on learning new skills and understanding the larger purpose of health care.* Expand your focus beyond one patient or one practice to the needs of a broader community.
4. *Assume positive intent.* Understand the rationale behind certain decisions that impact your own medical practice, even if you disagree, and then try to positively implement them.
5. *Express gratitude for the organization's willingness to invest in the professional growth of young physicians.* If the hospital is willing to invest time and money in their professional growth, that means you are viewed as a trusted future leader. Understand that this is a potent form of recognition.
6. *Don't let cynicism take over.* Keep a neutral mindset. Disillusionment can creep up very quickly when one sees colleagues moving on or a valued nurse being let go. All of us face challenging leadership decisions during our careers. Lean in.
7. *Refuse to distance yourself as a physician when decisions go contrary to your own thinking.* Stay at the decision-making table, even when it gets tough or discouraging. Dig deep into your resiliency, as you will need it as you grow in your leadership journey. No one said it would be easy! I agree with Angood when he writes:

    > Physician leaders with the right management skills have a distinct advantage over other business professionals in steering organizations toward providing high-quality yet cost-effective care, an idea that is supported by the fact that the best-performing hospitals, such as the Mayo Clinic, are largely physician-driven.[71]

And there you go. The leadership journey has already subtly started.

What Kind of Young Physician Leaders Do We Need?

Physician leadership is critical if we are to shepherd health care into a better future. Physicians have the skills, the experience, and the will to create a delivery system grounded in better health at lower costs. No wonder, then, that physician leaders have been described as "interface professionals" who bridge medicine and management, connecting an organization's front lines of care with related operational management, leadership, and governance.[72]

What, then, are the core competencies required for young physicians who may be pondering a future as a CMO or who are already aspiring to such a position? Countless subject matter experts have weighed in on this question. Consider just a few of them.

> *Peter B. Angood, MD*: Successful physician leaders need expertise in key competencies, including technical knowledge and skills, industry knowledge, problem-solving skills, emotional intelligence, communication, and commitment to lifelong learning.[73]
>
> *Bruce Spurlock, MD*: Successful leaders can embrace the idea that it's about creating a bigger vision rather than being precise and right on every decision. You have to be decisive. You're trained to be decisive, and that means getting rid of cognitive dissonance. The doctors who are most able to deal with cognitive dissonance, uncertainty, and ambiguity are the ones who can succeed.
>
> Successful leaders are in continual "learning mode." Physicians who move things forward in whatever they do are leaders—whether they are working from a recognized leadership position or not. When they take responsibility for making change happen, they're leaders. That can be at micro levels, it can be at macro levels, it can be over an entire health system, or one office; but the instant they take responsibility and

ownership, and have the drive to make things better, they become leaders. We need an army of those kinds of leaders to make a difference in healthcare. We need thousands and thousands of people just like that to improve the healthcare system.[74]

Charles Falcone, MD: By and large, there's not a lot of teamwork or collaborative skills taught in [the typical medical school or residency] environment. Many physicians have trouble working in the more collaborative team-based leadership models. As an executive recruiter, I try to assess that ability when we're placing senior physician executives these days and when we think about some of the traits, some of the soft skills that drive success beyond the classic skills of understanding how operations work or financial acumen.[75]

Jason Petros, deputy managing partner of health care for Witt-Kieffer in Chicago: In day-to-day practice, physicians are typically accustomed to a more autonomous, hierarchal focus—they're not necessarily team players. But as CEO, a physician must be able to inspire and empower others to get the job done. The lone wolf physician leader is not a paradigm that will work.[76]

Maureen Bisognano, president emerita and senior fellow of the Institute for Healthcare Improvement: Many physicians . . . make the mistake of assuming clinical skill translates into leadership ability. The two do not always go hand in hand. Clinical skills are certainly a requirement, but they are not enough. It's about vision and strategy and moving a system culturally toward the "Triple Aim" of better health, better care, and lower cost. That's very different from solving problems one at a time. It requires a different tempo of decision-making, a different scope of work and a different set of skills.[77]

I agree with Michael J. Menen, MD, that "a CMO should have a record of effectively leading and managing teams. The importance of strong interpersonal skills and the ability to build relationships with both internal and external stakeholders cannot be overstated. CMOs must be able to effectively communicate with various stakeholders, including executives, regulators, and policymakers. The ability to clearly articulate complex medical concepts and describe a compelling vision is essential in driving positive change within the organization."[78]

Additionally, CMOs must learn how to lead through influence more than through a traditional hierarchy. They must become diplomats who collaborate effectively with various stakeholders, relying a great deal on their abilities to persuade and negotiate fairly. Persuading and negotiating like a seasoned diplomat is an important—or maybe I should say crucial—part of the job. Again, I appreciate what Dr. Menen has to say:

> The ability to collaborate effectively with other departments is crucial for the overall success and effectiveness of the organization and the CMO. Even if a CMO and other leaders have the same goals, compromises often are necessary to realize initiatives and to meet the organization's overall goals.
>
> Each department brings its unique perspective, expertise, and resources to the table. Only by understanding what motivates different departments can a CMO organize a consensus and develop integrated solutions that will meet the needs of all stakeholders. Sharing resources between departments reduces redundancies and streamlines tasks.[79]

While I will expand on these required characteristics in part 3, for now I'll say that successful physician leaders must demonstrate technical knowledge, industry expertise, problem-solving abilities, emotional intelligence, strong communication, and a dedication to ongoing learning.

Don't worry if you're thinking to yourself, *But I don't possess some of those characteristics!* That observation was certainly true of me when I began my own physician leadership journey several years ago. Thankfully, though, what you may not have *right now*, you can acquire along the way. Every one of the traits I just listed can be learned. If they couldn't be, I wouldn't be where I am right now.

Requirements for Preparation

What steps should an aspiring physician undertake to become adequately prepared for this role? First, you'll need to build on the courage you already have. The journey ahead is similar to a board examination. And how did you prepare for *that*? You read, you attended board prep meetings . . . and then you took the plunge.

Consider what follows as something of a leadership preparation checklist, but keep in mind that it's really just a start. Throughout this book, you will find material that describes the role in more detail. I hope that you may discover valuable insights that inspire your curiosity and motivate you on this critically important journey.

Leadership Preparation Checklist

1. *Gain medical knowledge.*

   Physicians must have ample reason to respect their leaders, and physician leaders who have more than fifteen years of bedside clinical care under their belts typically engender just that kind of respect. They can also give young physicians valuable insight from their firsthand experience. Amassing a sufficient amount of clinical bedside experience is crucial for anyone who wishes to take on the responsibilities of a CMO.

   According to Glenn Lux, MD, the CEO of Allegro Pediatrics, physician leaders are more likely to empathize with the demands of their colleagues' clinical responsibilities and to make decisions sensitive to their needs. Why? Because they speak the same language and share common histories with most types of clinicians. "We understand the soul of the business because we've done it," Lux said.[80]

2. *Invest in yourself.*

   Earning an additional master's degree beyond your MD/DO makes you a more marketable candidate. It not only enhances your résumé, but it also expands your horizons in medicine beyond clinical care. In addition, it shows your organization that you are interested, motivated, and eager to grow professionally.

   Of course, merely having an additional degree isn't enough. Elise MacCarroll-Wright, the president and CEO of a hospital in Illinois, says that "a lot of physicians are going back to school for their master's in business. Once they get their master's in business, they think they're ready to be a CMO. They think, *I have my master's, I'm a physician, I'm a leader—I want to be a chief medical officer.* They may be the most outstanding clinician; they may be their department's director with the ability to lead their department or specific service line; they might be clinically respected—but they need to have the required strategic mind. They must understand how to help run the *business* of health care."[81]

3. *Take leadership courses.*

   Expanding your leadership knowledge gives you a new vocabulary that will be needed when interacting with administrative leadership. Since most individuals in the C-suite don't understand medical terminology, you will have to master terms such as "budget neutral" or "offset cost." This mirrors what you already do when you find yourself trying to explain a diagnosis to a patient. In that case, you find appropriate nonmedical words to approximate the technical medical jargon.

And who might your future administrative colleagues be? They might include public officials, regulators, or legislators. In addition, as a CMO, you will be expected to speak effectively to community members and to know how to engage with them in productive ways.

Mark Goldberger, a cardiologist at Maimonides Cardiology in New York City, insists that "leadership in 2025 requires individuals who are skilled in managing healthcare institutions and have expertise in non-medical areas such as management, IT, AI, public policy, etc."[82]

4. *Enhance your emotional intelligence.*

   Unlike our IQ, which is a static number, we can enhance our EQ because it's a learned skill (see chapter 7). For most of us as physicians, this is a whole new muscle that we must continually strengthen. Leadership IQ is applied approximately 20 percent of the time, while outcomes are influenced primarily by emotional intelligence.

   Grace Terrell, MD, says that although several qualities are required to make someone a great physician leader, one of the most important is the ability to listen and to have perspective above and beyond one's own point of view. She says it's crucial to understand the limitations of the skill set you bring to a leadership position, to recognize the wisdom of learning from others, and to put in the time it takes to learn how to work as part of a team.[83]

5. *Learn to work in a team.*

   This is not a new concept for physicians. Some specialties, such as proceduralist work, require effective teamwork. But there is a significant difference as you prepare for the CMO role: You must realize that you might not automatically be the leader of the team. In the administrative space of leadership, the team concept is not hierarchical.

In addition to the five critical areas just mentioned, you'll need to acquire other skill sets to become an effective CMO. The American Association of Physician Leadership lists the following important leadership traits and characteristics for any CMO: self-management, professional capabilities, team building and teamwork, problem-solving, motivations and thinking style, operations and policy, quality and risk, finance, and strategy and innovation.[84] It also lists seven traits that it believes cover the major attributes of leadership: adaptable, ethical, visionary, introspective, vigilant, tactical, and knowledgeable.[85]

Sean Higginson, the chief of radiology at Augusta Medical Group in Fishersville, Georgia, said that "U.S. healthcare desperately needs more experienced physician leaders. . . . The best physician leaders are ones that not only have expertise managing their own domain but can break out of the silo and effectively anticipate the perspectives of the other stakeholders in a health system."[86]

Brian Neal, the attending physician of Huntington Hospital and the South Shore Emergency Department of Northwell Health in Huntington, New York, said, "Physician leadership must always begin with the patient at its core. . . . Effective leadership entails fostering cohesion and respect among all members involved in patient care—nurses, technicians, radiologists, consultants and fellow physicians—working collaboratively at the bedside. Anchoring leadership in these core principles of medicine allows physicians to focus on what truly matters, despite the growing administrative burdens, staffing challenges, and the increasingly complex medico-legal environment. By centering leadership on patient care and team collaboration, physicians can navigate and transcend these external pressures."[87]

Does all that sound like a big challenge? It should, because it is! Having said that, I can testify that the rewards *far* outstrip anything else I've ever known.

Begin *Now* to Prepare for Your Leadership Future

I recommend a two-step process to begin preparing for your leadership future. First, find a mentor. Second, ask your organization to invest in you with a coach—and yes, mentors differ from coaches.

While mentoring is a long-term *relationship* aimed at personal and professional development, coaching is typically short-term and goal-oriented. Coaches work with individuals to improve specific skills or achieve designated outcomes, often using structured sessions to facilitate the process.

Former hospital CEO Ken Lukhard declared, "Great doctors find great doctors, recruit them, mentor them, and launch them, and then they go on to do great things. I'm just totally sold on the idea. I mentored many of my CMOs, but clearly *not* on how to be a brilliant scientist or how to apply that in an organization. My mentoring was around core leadership skills—how to lead a meeting, how to listen to people, how to tactfully not let somebody dominate a meeting and redirect them instead. You have to draw the people into a conversation. My mentoring was very much around leadership."

Charles Falcone, MD, said, "I would encourage physician leaders to understand what it is they enjoy, then set a course for how they want to get there. Find a mentor who is skilled in helping them think through the pathway and what's open and available for physician leaders, especially in their early times of wanting to make that transition. One of the hardest things for physicians is making that transition from clinical to executive. I would encourage them to talk to folks like me or other leaders in the industry to get a sense of how others have become successful. I would encourage them to be open-minded about opportunities that arise, especially regarding entry-level positions within systems." Falcone added that he's a "big advocate" of finding mentors outside of the physician's institutions.[88]

I've observed that most young leaders take offense to critical feedback. But if they have a mentor in their corner—a battle buddy, a more mature leader—then they have someone to bounce their frustrations off of and perhaps heed counsel from. When these young leaders finally ask, "What do you think?" a mature leader has enough experience and insight to reply, "Hmmm, well, it sounds as though he's right. Maybe that conversation could have gone a little differently. What might have happened if you had said *this*?"

As you grow in emotional intelligence, you won't always need someone else to help you see the real problem. In time, you'll gain the insight to say to yourself, "I could have saved myself a lot of grief and time if I had done *this* instead." Eventually, you learn how to stave off those confrontations before they happen and yet still arrive at an answer or resolution to which everyone can say, "Yes, I think that will work."

We all need to be willing to be vulnerable to mentors, executive coaches, or other coaches. We need to embrace the insight they offer and say, "Yeah, I need to listen more. I need to build that skill."

Peer coaching is widely recognized as an important strategy for physician leadership and well-being. As we know, physicians tend to listen to their peers more than to anyone else. Such listening contributes to resilience.

Early in my career, I felt really troubled about a difficult intubation; the thought of causing a patient harm was very difficult for me to fathom. At lunch hour in the physician lounge one day, a pulmonologist noticed my downcast demeanor and asked if I was doing okay. It was just the opening that I needed at that time. We shared both professional and personal anecdotes. The ten-minute conversation provided me with a much-needed sense of relief. I remember those moments clearly and can still visualize the lunchroom.

I believe peer conversations are the best way to build resiliency and morale. So, find a peer that you trust and make them your battle buddy. Collaboration is essential, and support should always be available. In my world, TEAM stands for Together, Everyone Achieves More.

What Can *You* Accomplish?

Do you know the best part of all this? The primary focus of every chief medical officer is precisely what physicians love most and are best skilled to do: enhance patient safety and deliver high-quality care.

Ken Lukhard sums it up well: "To improve clinical services, to develop and implement quality improvement at its core, to enhance key clinical metrics—that whole area of health, of hospital functioning—I believe it all rests on the shoulders of the CMO. A good CMO takes you to the promised land, while a bad one gets you lost and wandering in the wilderness, looking for the right way to get out of there. If you hire the right one, if you get the right one in place, it launches the organization."

So, here's my advice: Keep growing, keep learning, and do your best to enjoy the ride. Each day will present unique circumstances and experiences.

Every now and then, someone asks if I regret being a CMO. I sometimes answer, "It depends on which day you ask." On most days, though, my unequivocal response is, "No."

The fact is that the need for physicians to serve as team builders, motivators, communicators, and change agents has grown exponentially. We live in an era that recognizes health care organizations far more for their medical performance than for their operational acumen. "As the complexities of healthcare reform take shape, more physicians will be called upon to lead the change," says John R. Combes, MD, chief communications and public policy officer for the Accreditation Council for Graduate Medical Education and a former senior vice president at the American Hospital Association. He asks, "Who better to address challenges faced by healthcare organizations today than those with experience on the front lines?"[89]

Should You Be One of Them?

Should you step into the world of health care leadership? No one can make this decision but you. But if you should say, "Yes, I want to go there" (and I hope you do), just realize it's not an easy road. It will require a lot of hard work. Still, neither of those things is a good reason for preventing you from moving forward.

Although lifelong learning is not a new concept for physicians, the timing of altering a professional career can sometimes be the determining factor in our decision-making (see chapter 9). In my early fifties, for example, I reached a crossroads. After more than twenty years in clinical medicine, I realized I probably had maybe fifteen years left to impact and improve health care safety before my retirement. *That* was my motivation for becoming a CMO. I needed to try to make a change.

I feel strongly that physicians make better health care leaders, but then again, I'm biased. It is my sincere hope that this book inspires you, motivates you, and provides you with the tools you need to succeed as a future chief medical officer.

May the force be with you!

What Future Do You Want to Create?

I'll end this chapter with a few wise words from two experienced CMOs.

When asked what the future holds for physician leadership in health care, the current president and CEO of Cynosure Health, Bruce Spurlock, MD, responded with enthusiasm: "I think the future for physician leaders [depends on] the future they want to create. The system is going to change in ways that we can't predict. . . . A lot of it's going to be creating what we think is the right future, and that's up to us."[90]

We are quickly moving into a period when physicians will have exceptional opportunities to provide excellent and innovative leadership. I sincerely hope that you will become one of those excellent and innovative leaders. We certainly need you!

One young physician with his sights firmly set on a future leadership role in health care told me something that I hope resonates with you. He said:

> Change is an inevitable yet exciting aspect of life, often ushering in a period of uncertainty. In medicine, where the landscape is constantly shifting due to evolving practices and technologies, this uncertainty can be especially overwhelming for physicians. New challenges—such as adapting to a new electronic medical record system, meeting new CMS requirements, incorporating updated billing codes, or mastering cutting-edge technologies like robotic systems for biopsies—are all part of the ever-changing demands of the field. After eighteen years of practice in my specialty, rather than becoming frustrated or overwhelmed, I have chosen to embrace these challenges head-on and take my career beyond individual patient care. Transitioning into a leadership role, such as chief medical officer, requires not only passion and motivation, but also a deep curiosity about improving the health care system on a broader scale—not just for physicians, but for hospital teams and the organization as a whole. Rather than seeing the evolving landscape of medicine as a burden, I view it as an opportunity to enhance patient care on a systemic level and drive positive change within the institutions I serve.[91]

If you feel even a tinge of what this young physician does, I urge you to seriously explore whether a CMO role might be right for you. Who knows what the future might bring?

PART 2

Who Needs a CMO?

The chief medical officer is an evolving, growing role, not only in hospitals but in organizations beyond hospitals. Even tech companies such as Microsoft and Google have realized its importance, especially as artificial intelligence becomes more prevalent throughout health care.

Who are the main stakeholders that benefit from having a CMO? First and foremost is any health care organization's medical staff. CMOs make the lives of their medical staff easier, safer, and more efficient. Therefore, every CMO must have a good, trusting relationship with both medical staff leadership and those in the trenches.

Second is an organization's CEO. The CMO must work closely with the CEO, the organization's authority figure, to enable the organization to fulfill the Quadruple Aim of health care. That means that each must have the other's back. The two must always remain aligned and in sync.

Finally, there are the patients, the members of the community whom we are so privileged to serve. The CMO plays an indispensable role in delivering safe, effective patient care.

4

WHY PHYSICIANS NEED A CMO

The overarching reason why physicians need a chief medical officer is one you've heard already: The CMO is the *only* clinical voice in the administrative corridor. CMOs are physicians themselves, with years of successful clinical experience under their belts. They have walked in the physicians' shoes, fought the physicians' battles, cared for patients, and found productive ways to work with administrators. Now, as administrators themselves, CMOs know how to represent the concerns of physicians in the administrative corridor. They understand the challenges unique to physicians, as well as the elements of the job that most appeal to medical personnel.

Beyond that broad scope, I believe that physicians need CMOs in at least eight specific areas, each of which we'll consider in turn:

1. Maintaining organizational alignment
2. Delivering high-quality care
3. Improving physician well-being
4. Preventing medical errors
5. Maintaining compliance with regulatory agencies
6. Providing a just culture peer review process
7. Building trust
8. Developing a pipeline for future physician leaders

In essence, effective CMOs help make the professional lives of physicians more efficient, manageable, and enjoyable. CMOs and physicians need each other.

Maintaining Organizational Alignment

Maintaining alignment between a hospital system and its medical staff is critical for the success of both, and the CMO is key to enabling such alignment.

Physicians rightfully pride themselves on providing the best possible patient-centric care. They take it personally when hospital metrics are negatively impacted. Hospital systems achieve high reliability and safe clinical operations *only* when physicians are aligned with the goals and strategies of the organization. Indeed, this happens most often when physicians take the lead. Hospital systems and physicians must work together to achieve success—and the CMO is central to this happening.

It has been my experience that medical staff appreciate having a physician leader with clinical expertise and leadership skills working in the C-suite. CMOs are bilingual, in a sense, in that they speak both "clinical" and "administrative." They can therefore translate in both directions, helping administrators to understand the concerns and challenges of physicians and helping physicians to understand and appreciate the imperatives and work of the administrators.

For these reasons, it is critical to have the CMO's clinical voice in administrative corridors. If no other reason existed for physicians needing a chief medical officer, this would be enough. But, of course, many other potent reasons also exist.

Delivering High-Quality Care

Josephine L. Young, MD, MPH, the medical director of Premera Blue Cross and formerly the chief operations officer for Allegro Pediatrics, claims that having medical colleagues in administrative leadership positions helps to ensure that a medical practice remains focused on what is best for patients rather than on what produces financial gain. She says that a blend of clinical and nonclinical backgrounds, including specialized expertise in information technology and finance, "allows you to treat the business side like a business and to draw from the best of both worlds."[92]

Most physicians in the trenches need guidance on nonclinical hospital issues. They need someone who has walked in their shoes to explain the "why" behind a nonclinical task. In the larger hospital setting, tasks that might seem mundane and non-patient-centric are nevertheless fundamental for the larger good. Since physicians tend to listen to their peers more than to nonclinical colleagues, a savvy CMO will have (or will choose to develop) the skill set required to translate the need for physician action and how that action will impact patient care.

Organizations such as CMS, the Leapfrog Group, and *U.S. News & World Report* publish physician and hospital data that is accessible in the public domain. These are not mutually exclusive but rather interdependent. This is the CMO's main message. The quality of care can improve only if hospitals and physicians are aligned. Health care infections, adverse events, and patient experience will not improve through the actions of one entity alone. All must be rowing in the same direction to elevate the care that is delivered to every patient, every time.

"Zero preventable harm" is not a slogan but rather a journey that all high reliability organizations have undertaken. This translates to no health care–associated conditions, such as CAUTI, CLABSI, and SSI. Collaborative processes led by the CMO are essential for reaching this goal.

Improving Physician Well-Being

CMOs play a vital role in supporting physician well-being. They have lived the disenchantment that their peers often feel with a constant barrage of administrative tasks. But physician well-being involves far more than successfully dealing with administrative burdens! An unsatisfactory sense of recognition and value is a major contributor to physician burnout. Physicians need to both *believe* and *feel* that they are valued and heard. Successful CMOs, therefore, create both a path and a mechanism for this to happen.

Physicians often underestimate how much responsibility they carry on their shoulders. Too often, they bring work home with them. If a patient dies, they don't "just get over it." And yet, while the trauma lives with them for a *very* long time, they rarely share the struggle with anybody. To help safeguard or improve their well-being, CMOs must provide two key things:

1. A peer infrastructure that provides physicians with the opportunity to talk to one another
2. Professional, anonymous counseling support

A high percentage of physicians feel weak when they seek help. A 2018 article published by the American Medical Association named five reasons why physicians are less likely than the general population to seek support. Many physicians do not reach out for help when stressed because they (1) fear licensure problems; (2) are constrained by the "physician personality" (i.e., doubt, guilt, an exaggerated sense of personal responsibility); (3) have been programmed to cope alone; (4) have a survival mentality (i.e., "I have to make it through this"); and (5) suffer from self-doubt and imposter syndrome.[93]

While I am grateful that this appears to be less of a stigma with the new generation of physician leaders, it nevertheless affects a large percentage of practicing physicians. In fact, such a refusal to seek help, or at least the hesitance to seek it, is known to prompt many physicians to retire early. One study found that 37 percent of physicians surveyed reported looking forward to retirement as an effective strategy for well-being.[94] Bruce Spurlock, MD, reports that burned-out physicians often tell him that they don't enjoy their profession as much as they used to, so they say, "I'm retiring at 59, 60, or 61 because it's just not there for me anymore—and besides, my retirement account is in good shape."[95]

How do we help valued physicians stay in the game a little longer? Many hospitals and health care organizations place a great deal of emphasis on what I'd call "event planning." But as one of my colleagues told me, "There is only so much yoga we can do to build resilience." For me, improving physicians' well-being begins with doing a better job of assessing their specific work challenges. We must ask, "How can we enhance the effectiveness of our well-being committees? How can we use these groups to positively impact the workflow for our physicians in the trenches?"

One glaring example immediately comes to mind. Physicians often receive a large volume of texts throughout their workday. At the same time, the most common cause for medical errors is interruption. Unnecessary texts tend to disrupt a physician's thought process, which can lead to errors—and those errors can significantly decrease a physician's sense of personal well-being.

In one hospital, we used our hospitalists to build and implement a process designed to decrease the number of texts from nurses to physicians. This required educating our nursing teams. Although it took some time, the number of texts dropped substantially. The reduction in text numbers positively influenced both physician well-being and patient care.

All physicians, without exception, want ease of practice. If we can figure out ways to make providing care less burdensome on them, we will find a cache of magic bullets. I believe artificial intelligence has helped us there recently (although I say this with trepidation. While AI has profound ramifications for ethical care, that is a discussion for another book.)

Technology has both benefits and drawbacks. For example, many changes have occurred recently in the way we manage electronic medical records (EMR), a great many of them due to technology. But at the same time, it has often been said that physicians retire when the EMR they're used to is replaced. Why? It's hard to learn a new system, and many senior physicians don't see learning that new system as worthwhile, so they retire.

As AI becomes increasingly integrated into EMR, many of us see great potential for technology to support clinicians in their work. I remember when AI was first integrated into our EMR. We had one superb physician on the verge of retirement. He could not bear to think of the upcoming EMR change. However, when the AI went live and his documentation immediately became much easier, he found himself with more time to spend with his patients, the very thing he'd been trained to do and what he felt passionate about. He therefore delayed his retirement by a few years, which was a *huge* win for us. We were able to retain an experienced, excellent physician who possessed a wealth of knowledge. Even more importantly, it was a huge win for our patients.

Every competent CMO must focus on physician wellness. Failure to do so can have catastrophic results. A recent article by Andrew Proulx, MD, published on the *Psychiatry Advisor* website, claimed that health care providers in the US "are facing what the CDC has classified as a mental health crisis. The AMA is focusing on early recognition of burnout and depression as common markers, factors, and comorbidities of suicidality."[96] The article quoted a 2022 statistic to claim that approximately 119 physicians die by suicide each year in the US. However, Proulx admitted that the number of physicians who die by suicide "is difficult to determine." The 119 annual suicide figure is based on extrapolating data from the CDC's National Violent Death Reporting System.[97]

The rate of death by suicide is higher for female physicians than for women in general. A study of about 1.84 million adult health care workers compared the rate of their fatal suicide attempts to non–health care professionals (HCPs). While the non-HCPs had a fatal suicide attempt rate of 12.6 per 100,000 individuals, health care support workers had a rate of 21.4, registered nurses a rate of 16.0, health technicians a rate of 15.6, and physicians a rate of 13.1.[98]

Another study published in February 2025 by *JAMA Psychiatry* noted that female physicians had higher rates of suicide than female nonphysicians in 2017, compared to male physicians and nonphysicians. The study also concluded that "compared to the general population and including all available jurisdiction data, physicians had higher odds of depressed mood as well as mental health and legal problems preceding suicide."[99] A retired physician commenting on the article stated that while "it is correctly noted that female physicians are more at risk for suicide than female non-physicians, the fact that male physicians are roughly twice as likely as female physicians to complete suicide is not even mentioned. I believe that both results are noteworthy."[100]

A 2020 survey conducted by the Physicians Foundation during the COVID-19 pandemic found that nearly one in four physicians (22 percent) knew a physician who had committed suicide during the pandemic, while the majority surveyed (58 percent of 2,334 respondents) expressed feelings of burnout (compared to 40 percent four years earlier).[101] In addition, the survey found that 18 percent of respondents reported an increased personal use of medications, alcohol, or illicit drugs; 37 percent said they wanted to retire the following year; and just 40 percent said their hospital or health system was "somewhat to very helpful" in their efforts aimed at increasing physician well-being.[102]

A different 2020 study predicted a national shortage of 139,160 physicians by 2030,[103] while a later projection by the National Center for Health Workforce Analysis forecast a deficit of 79,080 physicians by the same year.[104] Regardless of the actual number, it's clear that a physician shortage is coming. And as helpful as groups such as the Advanced Practice Partners can be,[105] their welcome efforts cannot fully resolve the problem. We need to develop additional ways to support the mental, physical, and spiritual health of our doctors. Keeping them intact is essential for providing quality clinical care. And once again, CMOs play an outsized role in working to maintain and improve physician well-being.

Preventing Medical Errors

Despite the release of the landmark book *To Err Is Human* two and a half decades ago, medical errors remain one of the top five reasons for patient harm. Medical errors, of course, often lead to lawsuits—and no clinician wants to find themselves in that situation. Medical care has become increasingly complex in today's highly litigious society.

The institution where I work is a high reliability organization, so it has a robust safety reporting system. We encourage our associates and clinicians to report any gap or opportunity that they identify, knowing they do so in a safe environment. In my capacity as CMO, I am responsible for evaluating all adverse events and implementing systems to effectively address any identified gaps. Our reporting system exists to improve care for the next patient who is in a similar situation to the previous patient.

Litigation is every physician's nightmare. Sometimes it is the last straw that pulls them toward retirement and away from clinical practice. Only a fellow physician, such as their CMO, truly understands the mental distress caused by being sued. It is essential for the chief medical officer to offer appropriate support to every physician experiencing such grief and to ensure measures are taken to prevent the occurrence of a "second victim" scenario. And such a scenario is not a myth; I have lived it. It undermines the physician's confidence and increases the likelihood of additional errors.

Now more than ever, our medical staff need a strong advocate in administrative leadership to express their concerns and implement systems to protect them medico-legally. Bad systems will outperform good clinicians any day! We need physician leaders to help establish good clinical systems. And who better to oversee such efforts than the CMO?

Maintaining Compliance with Regulatory Agencies

The director of quality at one health care organization explained that the CMO's support is vital for translating quality, safety, and regulatory priorities to physicians. She said the CMO also must make that communication more impactful, thus ensuring compliance with standards. She highlighted key metrics, such as readmission rates, mortality, safety of care, and patient experience, each of which requires physician involvement to achieve high standards.

Both hospital and physician metrics are in the public domain. Anyone can easily look them up to see how a specific hospital or physician rates. Someone seeking a new doctor can quickly check the physician's rating; they can also write their own reviews of the physician's and the hospital's performance on various websites. Many organizations look up health grades, while others widely publish the positive grades they find. The stress on physicians for maintaining such standards and for trying to generate positive patient reviews is unique in modern medicine. Such stress did not exist fifteen years ago.

I maintain that physicians are not taught *nearly* enough during their training about the oversight of their clinical delivery by various federal and state regulatory agencies. Certain organizations are "deemed" by CMS to regulate the delivery of health care. I have had the opportunity to work with both DNV Healthcare USA and the Joint Commission (as two of these "deemed organizations"). The due diligence exercised by such agencies is important and helps hospitals deliver safe care.

Physicians as a group strive to provide safe, high-quality care. They also have a desire to serve as clinical leaders. But medical jargon, like any jargon specific to various industries or specialized fields, often fails to communicate effectively to individuals not immersed in those industries or fields. Medical jargon, while it provides physicians with a shorthand way to quickly relay information to colleagues, often fails to meet regulatory and CMS requirements. The CMO ensures that physicians maintain accurate, timely documentation, both for their own compliance and for medico-legal safety.

The oft-repeated adage "Not documented, not done" is even more relevant today due to compliance requirements. If a physician documents that a patient has a urinary tract infection but does not accurately document that the infection was present on admission, this infection is labeled "hospital-acquired," thus impacting the complication rate or mortality rate associated with the physician(s) involved.

I've learned that there's a distinction to be made between "accurate" and "appropriate" documentation. The former is taught in med school—how to take an accurate history, how to correctly document the physical examination, and how to write a pristine SOAP note. The latter, however, presents challenges for us. For a multitude of reasons, physicians tend to document in ways that might implicate their own colleagues or hospital. I have received calls from Risk Management and Compliance regarding a physician's note stating, "Surgery is delayed due to understaffed OR" or "Anesthesia is unavailable." While these may seem to be correct descriptions to a physician unaware of the full situation, such documentation is referred to in some circles as a "chart war." Engaging in a full-scale chart war is not appropriate and does not serve any constructive purpose. Such documentation puts both the physicians and the hospital in regulatory jeopardy. It is a CMO's duty to help physicians understand that such chart wars are in no one's best interest, including their own.

If physicians believe that such an action decreases their own legal exposure, they have landed very far from the truth. Instead, it only implicates them further and makes any malpractice attorney's job much easier. This is the most crucial intervention that a CMO can engage in; it prevents unnecessary litigation harm for both physicians and the organization.

Another aspect of compliance is following policies and procedures. Such safeguards are in place for a reason. The quality director quoted earlier noted that surveyors may observe time-out procedures during regulatory surveys and that consistent high-quality performance is required to meet standards. This is just one small example of how the CMO helps maintain regulatory compliance for both physicians and hospitals.

Providing a Just Culture Peer Review Process

While medical staff generally monitor themselves effectively, this, too, depends on the leadership engagement of the medical executive committee. I have been privileged to work with good medical staff presidents who have partnered with me in developing and implementing a just peer review process.

It is not easy to do a face-to-face peer review of your own colleague with whom you may be going out for dinner later that same day! It is important that a CMO provides the proper tools for members of a peer review committee, as well as helps them build the required skill set to approach every case objectively and with a standardized process. I have helped build and establish a nonpunitive just culture peer review mechanism to do exactly that. What we built took the burden off physicians' shoulders when questioning their colleagues. Instead, it placed that burden squarely on the algorithm that we created. This made it easier for the physicians to do their job and identify gaps in care or processes that could be addressed for the next patient under our care.

One of the CEOs I worked with recognized the value of a CMO leading an efficient just peer review system, saying, "Having those peer-to-peers comes in handy. [The CMO will] do a deep dive, a kind of forensic review of the care that was delivered. So, she tries to head it off at the pass [i.e., the medical error] and keep it from happening again."

Physicians tend to err on the side of normalizing an event, while at other times (usually unknown to them), bias creeps in. It is the role of the CMO to guide and keep the peer review objective and unbiased. Physicians should feel secure reporting their peers' possible errors and be empowered to make tough decisions, such as limiting privileges or imposing suspensions.

I once called the medical staff president at one of my campuses to share the reasons for the summary suspension of a physician. Such a provision is included in all medical staff bylaws, serving as a fundamental guide for the governance of medical staff. This measure is used *only* when a physician poses a safety risk to another associate on campus. It requires the CEO, the CMO, and the medical staff president to be fully engaged and aligned. I vividly remember making the call to report the findings of our investigation. Medical staff leadership, the hospital CEO, human resources, and the legal team all coordinated closely, all of them relying on me, the CMO, for direction and execution. Our process safeguarded the hospital, the physician, and the medical staff.

Building Trust

I began this chapter by highlighting the necessary alignment between medical staff and hospital administration, which can happen only in the presence of a strong foundation of trust. But such trust must be earned both ways. The CMO plays a huge role in facilitating an environment of psychological safety in which physicians can freely express their concerns. Both the hospital and its medical staff aim to deliver safe, high-quality care to the community, but this is impossible to pull off without first building a secure foundation of trust.

Consider contracts, for example. Contracts often involve difficult conversations. In these negotiations, the CMO must work closely with the physician group and the CFO to find a win-win resolution. The process of coming to this resolution can either build or break trust. Regarding the difficult work of negotiating contracts, the CFO at one organization said of the CMO, "She does all this pre-work whenever we're dealing with conversations about positions. She works behind the scenes, sharing information with physicians so they're more receptive when we meet them. We know where our pain points are, and it's been a great partnership. It takes time and the skill of a talented CMO to get the contract negotiated and signed."[106]

A CMO ensures that quality indicators appear in every contract. Nonclinical staff cannot identify these, nor can they ensure alignment with organizational goals while maintaining compliance with various Stark regulations. (The federal Stark law prohibits physicians from referring Medicare patients to providers with whom they have a financial relationship, thus avoiding a conflict of interest.)

What quality metrics should a CMO emphasize? That depends on what kind of hospital the CMO is leading. A critical access hospital, for example, will have different needs than a comprehensive, stroke-certified level 1 trauma center. The CMO will have to guide participants to reach a workable agreement while continually respecting the identity and culture of the various groups involved. Is that difficult? It can be. But if we keep our focus on patient care, we will rarely go wrong.

Developing a Pipeline for Future Physician Leaders

With the demand for physician leaders continually growing, every CMO must learn how to develop a pipeline of physician talent. This takes deliberate, intentional steps and many years to build.

It doesn't matter much whether the medical staff is predominantly employed or independent. While it certainly makes the job easier if it is the former (mostly regarding change management), it has *no* effect on the quality of care delivered. Never forget that most physicians are passionate about quality for *their* patients, *their* way only.

As the CMO, you will have to curate the rough diamonds and train them on high reliability principles. That can be quite a difficult task, since personal accountability and high reliability pillars are foreign concepts to many physicians.

In my last hospital, we did an analysis of our medical staff and found that less than 40 percent of our physicians were under forty years old. We had an aging medical staff, and our need for a physician leader pipeline was clear. So, what did we do? We began a physician leadership institute and started tapping young talent to serve on various hospital committees. We implemented a physician recognition program that identified and acknowledged potential new leaders at multiple venues, both locally and across the company. We saw it as essential to expose our physician leaders to the mission of our organization.

I held many one-on-one sessions with future medical staff presidents, encouraging each of them to self-invest (see chapter 8). I shared my own experience and described the wide variety of certifications they could obtain. I also launched a newsletter targeting physicians as the primary audience. We highlighted all the good work that we saw happening on our campuses and publicly celebrated our wins. This approach helped sustain our physicians' engagement and enthusiasm for their work. The CFO with whom I collaborated on this venture expressed his appreciation for the newsletter:

> Another piece was epic during the big transition we went through in October of '23. She, of course, spearheaded with the physicians, ensuring that they got the training done. She offers tips every month in her monthly newsletter. That's the first time I've seen anybody do that. She puts in there all the information about happenings on the campus and in the C-suite, as well as what the administrative halls are doing about it. She also has engagement messages and makes it easy for docs to access them. She even shares global health advocacy, CMS regulation changes, and tips to maintain their license. All in one single place! It was a well-read campus newsletter that even I, as a CFO, looked forward to every month. This is yet another way she has developed to keep in touch with the medical staff.

It is *so* important for the CMO and the medical staff to remain connected at all times! I rarely miss a call from another physician, irrespective of day or time. I know that when a physician calls me, it is to share a patient safety gap. I respect their time by never missing their calls. I want to remain in touch.

This is how my organization intends to build a deep physician leadership pipeline that exists long after I move on to another role. This is what makes me so proud of what we have accomplished together so far—the CMO and medical staff working together with one goal at the forefront of everything: safe, high-quality care.

A Gratifying Role

CMOs help deliver high-quality care by translating administrative priorities into clinical practice, by supporting physician well-being through addressing burnout, and by preventing medical errors through safety initiatives. It is a gratifying role, as it directly impacts the well-being of the patients, physicians, and the organization itself.

5

WHY PATIENTS NEED A CMO

Three central desires beat in the heart of every patient who enters a hospital or medical facility to receive care. Our patients may not always speak their wishes out loud, but their urgent pleas always remain the same:

Don't harm me.

Heal me.

Be kind to me.

Patients come under our care in the most vulnerable phases of their lives. Their bodies are sick or broken or malfunctioning, and all they want subconsciously are these three things.

What is the CMO's role here? To ensure that physicians and team members in the trenches have the skill sets to avoid harming our patients, to heal them, and to be kind to them.

We in the medical community, of course, probably would not use the phrases "Don't harm," "Heal," and "Be kind" to describe our approach to health care. It is much more likely that we'd use the term "quality" to refer to the sum of these three pleas. And what do we mean by quality? As of March 2026, the World Health Organization (WHO) has defined quality of care on its website as "the degree to which health services for individuals and populations increase the likelihood of desired health outcomes."[107] The WHO further states that the quality health services we provide should be:

- *Safe*: We work to avoid causing harm to the individuals for whom the care is intended.
- *Effective*: We provide evidence-based health care services to those who need them.
- *Patient-centered*: We deliver care that responds to individual preferences, needs, and values.

The father of modern quality, W. Edwards Deming, once wrote that "it is not enough to do your best; you must know what to do, and *then* do your best."

Do these statements resonate with you? I hope so, because they describe the skill set and role of a physician leader—and there is *no one* more central to enhancing the safe, effective, patient-centered delivery of health care than the chief medical officer.

Let's take a look at these three key elements and the central role of the CMO in each of these domains.

Safe Delivery of Care

No other C-suite role is more focused on the safe delivery of care than the CMO. While the CEO oversees the operations of the hospital, the CFO focuses on EBIDTA targets, and the CNO monitors hourly productivity, the CMO is *solely* responsible for quality and patient safety. CMOs ensure a hospital's quality and patient safety in several ways.

Improving Safety Through Dyads

A chief medical officer shapes patient care through a collaborative decision-making model. A recent white paper published in *MDA Leadership* describes the value of dyads for improved health care leadership. Its executive summary states, "To help ensure continuing high-quality medical care and ongoing business success within a rapidly changing healthcare industry, many organizations are employing healthcare dyads—formal leadership partnerships between respected physician leaders and skilled administrators—to capitalize on the strengths and attributes of each."[108]

Although both administrators and CMOs work to establish (and are guided by) an organization's mission/vision/values, the CMO focuses on maintaining and improving the quality of clinical professionals, while health care administrators oversee day-to-day operations. Although both groups work on strategy, the CMO focuses on provider behaviors while the administrator focuses on practice management. Although both groups work to improve organizational culture, the CMO focuses on provider production while the administrator focuses on performance reporting. Although both work to improve overall performance, the CMO focuses on clinical innovation while the administrator focuses on supply chain issues. You get the idea. CMOs, working in tandem with appropriate health care administrators, can profoundly help improve an organization's safety performance.

The growing phenomenon of dyad leadership is relatively new but already has proven indispensable in health care institutions. The white paper quoted above explains why:

> With massive, paradigm-shifting transformation happening in healthcare, such as the transition to value-based payments under the Medicare Access and CHIP Reauthorization Act (MACRA), all physicians—and the administrators who work with and support them—will need to adapt to new business and leadership demands.[109]

MDA Leadership CEO Scott Nelson further explained that fluctuating "reimbursement dynamics and an aging population requiring more comprehensive care are challenging healthcare leaders to think very differently in terms of effectively delivering healthcare. Quality healthcare leadership means figuring out how do you offer the best possible care, as close to the patient as possible, and as affordably as possible. That's a conversation tailor-made for dyad leaders to address."[110]

Set Clear Safety Standards

In 2003, the Joint Commission established a quality and patient safety improvement program called the National Patient Safety Goals (NPSGs). The NPSGs help accredited organizations address specific areas of concern regarding patient safety. For 2025, the Joint Commission established the following eight National Patient Safety goals, intended to enhance patient safety in various health care settings.[111]

1. *Identify patients correctly.*

   Clinicians are to identify patients in at least two ways (e.g., their name and date of birth) to ensure that each patient receives the correct medication and treatment. During the COVID year, I learned that one of our physicians requested a bedside laryngoscopy but provided only the room number. The nurse did not ask for clarification through the safety check mechanism of reading back the telephone order. Meanwhile, the intended patient was moved to another room. Do you see the Swiss cheese aligning? The procedure was performed on the wrong patient.

   These safety check goals were developed for a reason. Following the high reliability pillar of integrity (see chapter 9) would have prevented the error.

2. *Improve staff communication.*

   Clinicians must ensure that important test results are communicated to the right staff on time. Every hospital has a critical lab value policy, whose main goal is to prevent patient harm by ensuring that providers are informed of critical test results in a timely manner. A safety event is just waiting to happen when the lab fails to connect with the bedside nurse, who might have difficulty connecting with the correct provider.

CMOs must regularly review this policy for effectiveness and maintain clear communication channels for frontline teams. Remember, most errors occur due to a lack of processes rather than individual failures.

3. *Use medicines safely.*

   Confirm medications are labelled accurately prior to procedures.

   Take extra care with patients on blood thinners.

   Record and pass along correct information about a patient's medicines.

   Capturing accurate medication history at the time of admission, as well as accurate medication reconciliation at discharge, are key to ensuring safe hospitalization for our patients. The CMO needs to work with nursing, pharmacy, and clinical informatics to ensure that effective education and processes are in place.

4. *Prevent infection.*

   Clinicians should implement hand hygiene guidelines from the Centers for Disease Control and Prevention or the WHO to reduce the risk of infections. I recently reviewed hand hygiene observation reports. As a next step, I made rounds on one unit to discuss with the staff their barriers to compliance. The common theme? Hand sanitizers were either not working or not located for easy access. I therefore collaborated with the Infection Prevention team and facilities to standardize sanitizers throughout the hospital. Such a straightforward solution can significantly affect hospital-acquired infection rates. Remember that poor processes will hamper good outcomes.

5. *Identify patient safety risks.*

   Clinicians should recognize and address specific risks to patient safety, including suicide risk.[112] This is a sentinel event and requires an RCA.

6. *Prevent mistakes in surgery.*

   Clinicians must ensure that the correct surgery is performed on the correct patient and at the correct site. This includes marking the surgical site and pausing before the procedure to confirm the details.

   A 2009 nonfiction book by Atul Gawande titled *The Checklist Manifesto: How to Get Things Right* focuses on the use of checklists in the business world and in the medical profession. The author examines how checklists can be used for greater efficiency, consistency, and safety. Gawande said he was inspired to write his book after reading a story about a young child who survived a fall into a frozen pond. He discovered that the physician who saved her life relied heavily on checklists. The book builds on and references the work done by the Safe Surgery Saves Lives study group, whose work was published in the *New England Journal of Medicine* in January 2009.

   Note that this goal has been in place for more than a decade, yet we *still* see wrong-site surgeries happening at an unacceptable rate in operating rooms across our country.

7. *Use alarms safely.*

   Health care organizations should improve the safety of alarm systems on medical equipment to ensure timely responses.[113] It is the CMO's responsibility to ensure our patients remain safe while hospitalized. A fall resulting in injury is a sentinel event requiring an RCA to identify gaps that can be addressed for the next patient we serve. Bed and chair alarms help prevent patient harm.

As CMO, I served on a falls committee and reviewed the link between benzodiazepine use and falls in geriatric patients. I then worked with the pharmacy, the process improvement team, and our physicians to develop and implement a policy that allowed our pharmacist to modify the dose for a benzo-naive patient after conferring with a physician. This action resulted in decreasing our rates of falls and patient harm.

8. *Improve health care equity.*

   Clinicians should identify health care disparities and develop plans to improve equity in patient care.[114] Maternal care disparities worldwide have been researched and validated. Disparities in health care exist in various domains, including race, ethnicity, gender, and underinsured/uninsured populations. Hospitals are therefore implementing processes to reduce such disparities. CMOs must spearhead this initiative in collaboration with quality and community partners. For nonprofit organizations, this will also impact the community needs assessment. The CMO is part of establishing this assessment, which impacts an organization's nonprofit status.

Starting January 1, 2026, the NPSGs will be replaced by the National Performance Goals (NPGs) established by the Joint Commission. They will focus on measurable, high-priority topics for health care settings. The transition to NPGs represents a significant shift in how health care organizations approach patient safety. By focusing on measurable outcomes and critical areas of care, these goals aim to enhance the overall safety and quality of health care services provided to patients.[115] CMOs must stay updated to maintain compliance and to consistently improve both patient safety and quality of care.

Effective Delivery of Health Care

Health care delivery is complex. It is effective when we ensure the quadruple aim is met—when high-quality care is delivered efficiently with good associate and physician satisfaction.[116]

Rounding with Other Executives

Chief medical officers, along with other executives, make patient rounds. It's a worthwhile exercise that allows patients to share feedback with executive leadership. I firmly believe the delivery of care will get better when we involve the patients and their families in the conversation.

Developing a Communication Plan to Improve Patient Safety

While doing research for this book, I found a compelling project focused on changing how clinical teams communicate.[117] A parent named Sharon Cray joined the advisory board of the Patient-Centered Outcomes Research Institute (PCORI) after her children were diagnosed with cystic fibrosis. She became a fierce advocate for patient safety. In time, she joined the advisory board of a PCORI-funded project aimed at improving communication among staff and parents in pediatric hospital units, with an eye toward reducing medical errors and, in turn, improving patient outcomes. One key component of the project was to empower parents—"lifting them out of the fog," as Cray described it—to be engaged in discussions about their children's care.

"You feel so helpless in a hospital, especially when your child is sick," Cray said. "To be involved in planning the care is empowering. It gives you direction."

Christopher Landrigan, MD, MPH, the chief of general pediatrics at Boston Children's Hospital, began investigating hospital communication dynamics more than a decade ago in hopes of reducing medical errors attributed to miscommunication. "We recognized that the ways doctors and nurses talked to each other were unstructured and prone to error," he said. Such observations were the impetus of what came to be called the I-PASS project. Landrigan's team standardized and bundled training elements as well as a written handoff process between doctors and nurses. As a result, investigators noticed an immediate reduction in medical errors that harmed patients.

I-PASS is an acronym for a structured, verbal communication plan employed during daily hospital rounds.

The **I** stands for "illness severity." The family involved reports whether a child was better, worse, or the same as the day before, with input from nurses.

The **P** stands for "patient summary." A brief summary of the patient's condition is supplied.

The **A** stands for "action list," which provides the main to-dos for the day.

The first **S** stands for "situation awareness and contingency planning." What should family and staff look out for, and what might happen?

The second **S** stands for "synthesis by receiver." The family reads back key points of the plan for the day.

This PCORI project applied training tools in an interdisciplinary way among doctors and nurses and integrated families' input during rounds (when the medical team meets to devise the day's care plan). The council provided practical tips, such as discouraging staff from using medical jargon to help families participate on an even footing. Alisa Khan, MD, MPH, a pediatric hospitalist who served as a project lead on the PCORI-funded study, wrote in an opinion piece in *The BMJ*, "On rounds, I ensure that the family's voice is heard first and last, and in their own words."

The PCORI research project tested I-PASS at seven hospitals, involving more than 150 doctors, nurses, and family members as co-investigators. The study found that harmful errors decreased by about 38 percent; patients had 46 percent fewer adverse events; and nurses and patients were more involved in rounds, with parents speaking up more and asking more questions.

The Institute for Patient and Family Centered Care (IPFCC) suggests that we can transform health care by more effectively engaging patients and families, but *how* we do so requires careful research. The Patient-Centered Outcomes Research Institute (PCORI defined engagement in research as "the meaningful involvement of patients, caregivers, clinicians, and other healthcare stakeholders (such as training institutions, payers, industry, policy makers) throughout the research process—from topic selection through design and conduct of research to dissemination of results."[118]

In one of our patient and family advisory councils, a family member of a cancer patient who had died some time before made a statement that really hit home. After losing a loved one, she said that others quickly moved on, leaving her isolated in her grief. Her comment generated several ideas, and as a result, a program was created that memorialized the name of the deceased and created a place for the family to grieve. A similar event at another hospital resulted in a garden for parents who lost newborns. Such initiatives strengthen the bond between caregivers and patients.

PCORI created a framework that presents a continuum for patients, family, and community stakeholders, from a low degree of involvement (being informed about a study) to the highest degree of involvement (directing and leading research studies).[119] The IPFCC promotes the use of patient and family advisors (PFAs) and patient and family advisory councils (PFACs) to bring a unique perspective and great value to research teams by sharing their expertise in:

- making decisions about health and health care,
- understanding their body's response to some condition or disease,
- deciding what care and treatments are right for them,
- determining their health goals,
- knowing what topics related to their condition or disease haven't been well researched,

- partnering with health care professionals to improve health care for others,
- collaborating across departments,
- maintaining clinical standards,
- improving patient flow,
- leading organizational change, and
- setting a clear vision.

This area of research has resulted in a high number of significant improvements in patient care.

The World Health Organization says that to fully realize the benefits of quality health care, health services must be *timely* and reduce waiting times, which sometimes can prove harmful. Waiting times and wait lists in health care are not mere inconveniences; they significantly affect health outcomes, equity, quality of care, and the efficiency of health systems, as well as citizen trust and confidence.[120] One closely followed metric is how many patients "left without being seen," a highly impactful number that directly impacts patient care. The CMO and the nearest clinical dyad CNO share direct responsibility for it. This system enables patients who visit our emergency rooms to be attended to in a timely and efficient manner. Picture a patient with chest pain leaving the ER because of delayed care. The potential for patient harm is enormous.

The World Health Organization states that health services must be *efficient*, which means maximizing the benefit of available resources and avoiding waste. Health care must deliver results (i.e., be effective) and reduce waste (i.e., be efficient). This is the basic difference between Six Sigma and the Lean process improvement theory. Lean primarily aims to eliminate waste and improve process flow, while Six Sigma focuses on reducing process variation and improving quality. The integration of both methodologies is known as Lean Six Sigma, which combines waste reduction with quality improvement. These methodologies can be used separately or together to improve operational efficiency in organizations. It is important for all CMOs to be well versed in both techniques as they lead change management.

For my own Lean Six Sigma Green Belt project, we used both the plan-do-study-act (PDSA) cycle and define, measure, analyze, improve, control (DMAIC) method to improve the process for osteoporosis screening rates, which were low in our resident clinic. Following implementation, osteoporosis screening rates increased within targeted patient groups. This was my first applied step toward preparing for the CMO role.

Patient-Centered Delivery of Care

Long gone are the days when some hospitals tended to treat patients like numbers, when the idea of "patient-centered care" was practically unheard of. And frankly, I'm grateful for that. Hospitals exist for the benefit of patients, not the other way around. The question for us is, how can CMOs improve a patient's experience in a health care facility? Let me outline a few of the more important ways.

Grievances and Concerns

Despite our best intentions and careful work, things go wrong, incidents happen, and mistakes get made. Such errors and adverse events often generate grievances and concerns from patients. We need to respond to these complaints in a timely way through a grid of patient-centered health care.

At the same time, we have a legal obligation to respond professionally. The response time for grievances and concerns can vary depending on the context and specific policies of each organization. Here are some general guidelines:[121]

- *Patient complaints*: Hospitals must respond to complaints concurrently while the patient is still hospitalized. This is the best time to do service recovery.

- *CMS grievance response time expectations*: Hospitals should respond to grievances within an average of seven days, with documentation of any delays and an estimated timeline for follow-up. Final resolution should occur within thirty days.

Time limits are crucial for maintaining patient trust and ensuring that grievances are addressed promptly and effectively. Organizations should implement systems to track and manage these time frames to ensure compliance and improve service quality.[122]

In a hospital where I used to work, the husband of a patient decided to put his wife in hospice. She died shortly thereafter, which caused him to struggle intensely with his decision. Multiple attempts had been made, both by the patient safety advocate and the medical director of the unit, to answer his anguished questions. Even the CEO sent a personal, handwritten letter, but none of these things helped him find closure. Finally, I called the widowed husband and had a meaningful conversation with him. I quickly realized that he was agonizing over his decision. He had no issues with our delivery of care; he simply needed to talk to a medical professional to share his feelings and to help him accept his decision, which had put him in agony.

CMOs are in a unique position to have such conversations, help bring closure to grieving relatives or friends, empathize with their feelings, and help them gain perspective on painful events.

Advance Directives: End-of-Life Discussions

Confusion often erupts when palliative care and hospice come up in discussion. It's possible you may have heard these terms used interchangeably, but palliative care and hospice are not the same.

Palliative and hospice care are different disciplines of medicine aimed at supporting people of all ages who are struggling with serious, long-term illnesses. Although these two forms of care are similar in some ways, they can differ as to when and where they are received and which treatment options are available.

Palliative care focuses on improving the quality of life for people with serious illnesses and their care partners. It is available to people of any age who need it, not just older adults. The major elements of palliative care include effectively managing a person's symptoms and ensuring that their care is coordinated. In addition to improving quality of life and helping with symptoms, palliative care can help patients understand their choices for medical treatment.

Hospice care also provides comprehensive comfort care as well as support for the family. The key difference in hospice is that all attempts to cure the person's illness are stopped. Hospice is provided for a person with a terminal illness whose life expectancy is less than six months. Hospice care is a specific type of palliative care provided in the final weeks or months of life.

Regardless of the illness, both palliative and hospice care share the same main goals:

- Improve quality of life.
- Increase overall comfort.
- Provide emotional support for the patient and their family.
- Help the patient make important decisions about their medical treatment.

Neither type of care requires a patient to give up their primary doctor. Both palliative and hospice care will work with a patient's primary doctor to coordinate and manage their care.

This topic is important to me, as I specialize in hospice and palliative care and have witnessed firsthand in my practice the effects of decisions in these areas. Patients often do not realize the critical nature of discussing their goals of care with their family members—and the age of the patient doesn't matter. I have had similar conversations countless times with patients of varied age groups. Young people often perceive mortality as a distant concept. But I often say, "Accidents happen, and none of us should leave the most important and difficult decisions for our loved ones who are grieving."

The treating physician is responsible for conducting challenging discussions, while the CMO is accountable for providing educational guidance to the medical staff in various venues. Examples include grand rounds focusing on advance directives, CME courses, and bioethics certifications. These are essential elements when leading an ethics committee or discussion.

In a former institution, I helped build a successful palliative care program. We assessed the program's success using metrics such as turnaround time for goals of care discussions, number of consultations, and timely hospice conversions, all aimed at benefiting both patients and their families. These are tough conversations that trained and empathetic individuals need to have with grieving individuals.

Disclosure of Adverse Events

The impact of the CMO is felt most deeply on patient care and medical staff education regarding the disclosure of adverse events. CMOs are trained to effectively handle the process of disclosure. There are two main reasons for this:

1. Disclosure helps a patient and their family to understand the loss they have just suffered.
2. Disclosure is a key step in their grief journey.

Disclosing adverse events to families is a critical aspect of patient care. It involves careful planning and thoughtful communication. Consider some key points about disclosing to families after an adverse event:[123]

- *Timing and context*: Disclose the event as soon as possible, ideally within sixty minutes after it is identified. This helps to maintain transparency and trust.
- *Team participation*: Involve all members of the clinical team, including the attending physician, in the initial conversation. This ensures a unified and compassionate approach.

- *Patient and family needs*: Assess the emotional and psychological needs of the patient and family and arrange for support, if necessary.
- *Communication techniques*: Use empathetic language, maintain eye contact, and avoid interrupting.
- *Follow-up*: After the initial disclosure, conduct a post-conversation huddle to debrief and discuss ongoing needs.

These steps are essential for creating a supportive environment and fostering a strong patient-facility relationship. According to a guideline published by the Risk Management Foundation of the Harvard Medical Institutions, Inc., "Above all, clinicians should be encouraged to express themselves as compassionate and caring human beings. Apply the 'Golden Rule:' What would you want to be told—and how would you want to be treated—if you were the patient or family? When in doubt, ask the patient and family if they are receiving the information they want and if their needs are being met."[124]

It is also important to address the emotional impact on health care practitioners, known as "second victims," and provide appropriate support for them.[125] At a hospital where I formerly worked, a complication occurred during heart surgery, leading to mortality. Two things immediately went through my mind. First, *how is the family?* And second, *how is the team doing*? The team included the surgeon, who serves as the team lead and who bears the maximum weight in such a tragic situation. I rushed over to the hospital to meet with the surgeon and the team to make sure they were all good. Clearly, the event had devastated them all. My job as CMO meant I needed to connect the dots between the surgeon and the anesthesiologist so that they were aligned in their thought processes. I wanted to ensure consensus on a clear message that would enable the family to obtain the information they required—and what they needed most was clarity, not confusion. I didn't want the family to hear the emotional reaction of distraught physicians and medical personnel.

Everybody was crying—every nurse, every OR tech, everyone in the room. I stayed with them late into the evening, talking to all of them. We also provided counseling afterward. The team faced a tough night and needed calm, objective leadership to stay safe.

At some point, this is all you can do. You must keep your emotions out of the situation, even as you work to control the emotions of every team member involved. That requires training and a lot of time.

Financial Implications

Physicians influence the quality of care and serve as financial stewards for both patients and the broader health care industry. This is where clinical documentation, coding, and utilization all intersect, with the CMO at the fulcrum.

Medicare has a rule that states a patient can be hospitalized either as an inpatient or an "outpatient with observation." Medicare A covers inpatient bills, while Medicare B covers physician bills. *Nothing* covers the outpatient observation (unless the patient has supplemental insurance). This means that if the patient is not assigned to the appropriate level of care, they might be negatively impacted financially.

The CMO role weighs in here. The CMO must educate physicians on documenting accurately to capture the most appropriate code. This is crucial because it affects both finances and regulatory compliance. We go into this in more detail in chapter 9.

The World Health Organization states that quality health care means providing services that are both *equitable* (i.e., providing care that does not vary in quality on account of the gender, ethnicity, geographic location, or socioeconomic status of the patient) and *integrated* (i.e., providing care that makes the full range of health services available throughout the patient's life course). CMOs have an impactful role in delivering both, which is another reason why patients need excellent CMOs.

The Importance of Medical Ethics

It would not be prudent to end this chapter without briefly discussing medical ethics. Medical ethics guide doctors, nurses, researchers, and policymakers to navigate complex situations. They also provide guidance on balancing scientific advancements with human values to deliver safe, high-quality care.

Modern medical ethics aregrounded on four key principles: autonomy, beneficence, non-maleficence, and justice. These principles serve as guiding pillars for ethical decision-making, helping health care professionals navigate complex situations while ensuring that patient rights, safety, and fairness remain at the core of medical practice and policy.

Autonomy refers to the patients' right to make their own health care decisions. In practice, autonomy is pivotal in cases such as making end-of-life decisions, refusing treatment, or selecting elective procedures. For example, a cancer patient may decline chemotherapy despite its potential benefits. Respecting autonomy means honoring this decision, even if the doctor personally disagrees.

Beneficence requires that health care providers act in the patient's best interest, promoting their well-being and positive outcomes. This goes beyond avoiding harm; it requires active efforts to do good, from recommending the most effective treatments to providing compassionate care. A doctor treating a stroke patient, for instance, might advocate for aggressive rehabilitation, understanding its long-term recovery benefits. In research, beneficence ensures that clinical trials serve the interests of participants and contribute to future medical progress.

Non-maleficence means "doing no harm." Health care providers must avoid causing unnecessary suffering, even when trying to help the patient. They should carefully weigh the potential risks and benefits of treatments and interventions to ensure ethical decision-making.

Justice in medical ethics ensures fairness in the distribution of health care resources, access to treatment, and decision-making. This principle requires that care be provided without discrimination, balancing individual needs with the broader societal context. In the case of organ transplants, for example, justice ensures recipients are chosen based on medical urgency rather than wealth or social status.

CMOs are tasked with making sure that their health care organization consistently upholds all four key principles. In this way, they serve as staunch advocates for patients who come to their hospital or clinic for care.

At one of my former hospitals, I founded an ethics committee to uphold professional standards and ensure ethical practices. It was a multidisciplinary group including physicians, nurses, chaplains, and ancillary team members. Case discussions involved inviting bioethicists to examine ethical principles and assist team members in navigating ethical dilemmas. The committee discussions assisted the care team members during difficult conversations, giving them appropriate words and guidance to take care of their patients and their families during their most difficult moments.

Do ethical dilemmas ever arise when conflicting moral principles make it difficult to know "the right thing to do?" Certainly. We saw it up close and personal during the peak of the pandemic. Common dilemmas include end-of-life decisions, patient confidentiality versus public safety, resource allocation, and informed consent challenges. Such situations require careful ethical reasoning to balance patients' rights and physicians' medical responsibility.

A good CMO confronts these dilemmas head-on, working collaboratively with colleagues to reach a "best for all" decision that reflects, as best as can be achieved, the principles of autonomy, beneficence, non-maleficence, and justice. And always—*always*—such a CMO hears the pleas of the patients who come for treatment:

Don't harm me.

Heal me.

Be kind to me.

And *that's* the bottom line of why all patients need a chief medical officer.

6

WHY HOSPITALS NEED A CMO

A strong CMO is the glue that keeps a hospital's medical staff functioning as a unit aligned with the organization's goals. The CMO clearly communicates the organization's patient safety and quality vision, so should we call the CMO the clinical CEO instead?

"If you don't have a strong medical staff," said Ken Lukhard, a retired hospital CEO, "and if you don't have a really strong, bright, and competent chief medical officer, you're starting the race a hundred yards behind everybody else. You *must* have great physician leadership. To me, that's just a must."

It doesn't stop there, of course. Listen to Lukhard again:

> The other thing you must have is a collegial and trusting relationship with the medical staff. As a CEO, if you don't have that, now you're not one hundred yards behind—now you're a *mile* behind the rest of the group starting the race. It's really built on the fulcrum of healthy, collaborative, and trusting relationships with physicians, because they're the key to the enterprise. They are the engine that makes it all work. I'm not discounting nurses—I love nurses, they're great—but they're not the clinical leaders of the organization. The clinical leaders are the physicians; they have to be. That's number one.

An effective CMO rallies a hospital's medical team to work together to achieve health care's Quadruple Aim of better patient care, improved health at a lower cost, and improved well-being. You could also think of the CMO as a health care organization's chief influencer, a professional who learns to work with all departments reporting to many different leaders, helping them to see the bigger picture and gain a higher understanding. All of this takes time and requires someone who knows how to lead with influence.

Patients First

Although the chief medical officer is a physician, he or she must consider the hospital's operations from all angles and perspectives. It's not "doctors first," or "nurses first," or "financial workers first," or "administrators first." If anyone's first, it's the patients—and to serve them well, everyone in the organization must work together for the common good. The CMO's job is to facilitate exactly that kind of active collaboration and cooperation.

The late Don Jernigan, the former president and CEO of the largest Protestant not-for-profit health care system in the United States, declared that early in his career, he observed "an organizational dichotomy. Our clinical people—nurses, doctors, and other clinicians—tended to look askance at our financial people, and vice versa. The two groups tolerated one another but considered each other deficient in some significant way."[126] Jernigan said he had "great fun" attacking "this diseased mindset." He'd get his clinical and financial people in the same room and, in a humorous way, reveal what they thought of each other. First, he turned to his medical personnel:

> You clinical people say, "We are the virtuous ones, the holy ones. We're the good people here. We're doing the Lord's work. We take care of sick people." And then you look over at these financial types and you say, "But we have this *other* group over here. They're really not very good people.

> They're money-grubbers, concerned only about the bottom line. They don't care about our patients, or about our mission, or about quality. They want us to make bricks without straw. They care only about finances—and some of that money is dirty."[127]

By then, his financial personnel had begun to snicker. But then came their turn:

> And here's what you financial people think about your clinical colleagues. You say, "These folks might be good people, but they're airheads. They don't have a clue about money or what it costs to do anything. They don't care if we run out of funds or even if we go bankrupt. They have no clue about how to effectively manage money, and they couldn't care less if they waste resources. They're all a few bricks short of a load."[128]

After he got everyone in the room laughing, Jernigan started educating them all on the concept of stewardship:

> This is crazy. I want financial people who care as much about the patients as the clinical people, and I want clinical people who have the skills and the knowledge to be good businesspeople. *And I will not tolerate you thinking ill of each other.* We are one team with one mission, and the attitudes that you sometimes express toward each other are inherently un-Christian. There are no good people or bad people in this organization. There are only two kinds of people here—good stewards or poor stewards.[129]

Effective CMOs share and even champion Jernigan's perspective. While they filter everything they do through a clinical mindset, their goal is to enable the hospital to thrive as it pursues health care's journey toward zero patient harm.

A chief financial officer at a Chicago-area health care system had this characteristic top of mind when asked to describe an "ideal" CMO: "They look at the job not just from the CMO side but from the hospital's side too. By that, I mean not only, 'I'm here to represent the physicians, the staff, and bring their issues to the C-suite to fix them,' but also to have multiple conversations that are not one-sided. They're willing to tell physicians, 'Well, here's the problem: The hospital is still not hitting budget, so your ask is a little too much. But if you come in at this level, there's an appetite for that. I agree that you need an increase, but you can't ask for this; there's no way. And I really want to see you get this increase.'"

This CFO declared that working with CMOs who act on behalf of both sides has been "a huge blessing. Where I came from before, it was all very one-sided. The only thing we heard was all the wants and all the things that *we* have to do to make *their* life better, at whatever cost. From a CFO perspective, that's not the answer. There must be some give and take and some win-win in this. Great CMOs excel the most right there. Their attitude is always a win-win." And then he offered an example of "splitting the difference" over some expense request:

> Our CMO usually brokers that. She'll say, "Guys, the hospital cannot afford to go there." And then she comes back to us and says, "We've got to give them *something*. How about 80/20 or 50/50?" She'll throw out these numbers. She knows they'll never agree to *that*, but she already knows they were probably going to agree to *this*. She's already planted the seed, with both them and us.

Effective CMOs often have such conversations outside of the boardroom, "maybe in the parking garage," the CFO said. "That is what I'm looking for, somebody who'll come in and not just bring all the problems, because we hear that already. We hear about it when a case doesn't go well or when somebody's mad about an anesthesiologist. They won't actually talk to that anesthesiologist; they'll talk to us and say, 'You have to do something about that anesthesiologist.' So, we get the CMO involved. We need somebody who comes in with that kind of an approach, a win-win, never 'us' against 'them.'"

One hospital's director of risk expressed a similar outlook, especially regarding a CMO being willing to have difficult conversations. "Some CMOs don't necessarily want to get their hands dirty," she said. "I need the CMO to have a conversation with a certain provider, but he seems hesitant to do so, or he tries to pass it on to someone else—even in those instances where I'd say, 'No, this needs to come from the chief medical officer.' Sometimes the CMO can get defensive or try to make excuses. With our event reporting system and complaints and grievances, at times you see patterns regarding some physicians that you just can't ignore. It *has* to be addressed. Maybe a doctor has a reputation for being difficult or not wanting to listen. Some CMOs don't want to have that conversation—but they're the chief medical officer! It's not just a title. They're the clinical administrator; they *have* to go and do this."

In my current role, I work as a regional CMO, focusing on the main campus but collaborating with part-time CMOs at four facilities. I must work at remaining totally aligned with all of them. We have monthly check-ins so that we can effectively regionalize our processes. The work of a regional CMO can get a bit complicated because the administration and leadership of the various system hospitals differ in many ways from one another. As the regional CMO, you must first understand the cultural nuances and then help break down those natural barriers, because although every C-suite has its own budget, together they function as a unified regional system.

From my perspective, it matters very little whether a stress test is done at Hospital A while a cardiac angiogram is done at Hospital B, but the decision does matter to the bottom lines of the affected campuses. So, the CEO of Hospital A will ask me, "Why did this patient go from this hospital to Hospital B? The procedure could have been done here." I might reply, "The choice came down to better patient care." The CEO may not agree, but he or she will listen. And that's the role of an effective CMO—to explain standardization, decrease variation, and clarify the "why" to administrative leadership and medical staff. Both must work together to ensure safe, high-quality patient care.

Six Reasons Why Hospitals Need CMOs

While hospitals need CMOs for countless reasons, let me highlight six of the most important.

1. Utilization management

How efficiently a hospital uses its resources impacts the finances of both the hospital and its patients. Poor utilization of resources can wreak havoc on a hospital's revenue cycle.

I've been a member of a value analysis team that looked at all the new supplies coming into the hospital. It was my role as the clinical leader in that group to explain in layman's terms what the new supplies meant and how a new approach would benefit both the hospital and patients. Questions would be asked of vendors, followed by a possible acknowledgment that their analysis was sound or that another option would be preferable. Sometimes I'd simply say, "We need this as we grow and to keep up with changes in medicine."

The CFO I quoted earlier said, "Whenever our CMO says anything like 'We need this,' it's an automatic 'yes' for me, because I trust that she has the best interest in mind of both the patient and the hospital. And that's been a blessing, to have somebody who will speak up on those issues. We all highly rely on her analysis of what the studies show or how those studies might not directly apply to our situation."

2. Clinical documentation

Appropriate documentation positively impacts value-based metrics and enables us to effectively manage critically ill patients. We have a clinical documentation integrity (CDI) program that reports up to this role. As the CMO, it is my responsibility to ensure that this program is compliant and optimized, as it impacts the publicly reported metrics for both the hospital and its physicians. The goal of this program is to capture the most accurate documentation, as the medical language is quite different from what is needed to code the chart.

It is the responsibility of the CMO to not only educate the staff in this department, but also to advise physicians on the "why" behind how they are asked to answer any clarifying queries. This alignment influences hospital revenue and ensures its physicians receive proper credit for patient care.

The optimization of this department also impacts the length of stay (LOS), a dreaded metric that all hospital systems follow. Physicians often say, "My patients are sicker than others," when discussing their own metrics. Because physicians typically concentrate on their own patients, it is the CMO's responsibility to provide the relevant data and facilitate understanding of the broader context. Physicians trust accurate data over the CMO's input; that's just the nature of the physician psyche. And only another physician who has lived in their shoes can fully understand it.

3. Appeals and denials

CMOs help to appeal coverage denials by insurance companies. We collaborate with the patient's physician to draft a letter to the insurance company appealing the denial. Physician advisors then have a phone conversation with the insurance company, which also has a medical director and a physician advisor. These physicians and administrators connect and then either deny or accept the appeal. Of course, their decisions have an impact on the hospital's revenue stream.

4. Care management

CMOs have a huge impact on patient care by ensuring that patients have an appropriate LOS in the hospital. Contrary to common belief, hospitals are *not* safe places to remain for extended periods. The longer a patient stays in a hospital, the higher the chances that some adverse event will occur (e.g., a fall, a drug reaction, an infection). It is the role of the CMO to explain this reality to both their physician colleagues and to patients.

An extended LOS not only uses more supplies but also demands additional staff time, meals, medications, and space. An effective CMO addresses key issues to boost hospital efficiency and profitability. Did you know that in 2022, US national health expenditures exceeded $4.4 *trillion*? That was 17.4 percent of the country's gross domestic product.[130]

Do you think optimizing LOS makes a difference? It does.

In many hospitals, a care management team reports directly to the CMO. That team typically includes nurses, social workers, and often physician advisors. The team's role is to ensure that the patient is hospitalized for the appropriate amount of time. Medicare (and now other insurance companies) pay by diagnosis-related group (DRG). Medicare assigns a fixed reimbursement to a specific diagnosis.

To illustrate: Suppose the hospital is reimbursed one hundred dollars for three days of hospitalization for a case of simple pneumonia. If that simple pneumonia patient stays for four or more days, those additional days are not reimbursed. Remember the clinical documentation team in the second bullet point? Here is how they intersect and impact LOS.

A clinical documentation specialist reviews the patient's medical record for physician documentation. Was it simple or complex pneumonia? The specialist then sends the query to the treating physician, and if the physician agrees, complex pneumonia is documented. This changes the DRG's length of stay from three to five days. If the physician disagrees, the CMO's job is to discuss the issue, clarify any confusion, and ensure proper documentation. This process greatly impacts the hospital's revenue stream to the tune of millions of dollars annually.

The CMO, together with the clinical documentation team, also impacts another key metric: mortality. This is a publicly reported metric that impacts 22 percent of the CMS star ratings. In partnership with the CNO at one of my previous hospitals, I helped establish a sepsis committee with just one goal: to decrease mortality rates for patients admitted in septic shock. We established a multidisciplinary team comprised of pharmacists, nurses, phlebotomists, respiratory care specialists, physicians, and additional specialists. In the end, our mortality rate for septic shock decreased by over 50 percent. Such a result does not take place unless the CMO walks in all lanes and intersects with leaders from all departments.

CMOs also empower care management department members to work together to build a safe transition plan once a patient is discharged. This protects patients and benefits both their finances and the hospital's. "Getting patients to stay the right amount of time in the hospital, especially the ED, had a huge, positive impact on patients, on the hospital, on our staff, and on our finances," one CFO told me. Placing individuals in the appropriate setting enables a more efficient transfer from the emergency department to inpatient units, helping to reduce pressure on ED resources. It also reduces waste.

With the shift to value-based purchasing and DRG payments, the CMO plays a vital role in guiding physicians to be effective financial stewards in addition to maintaining their clinical expertise. The CMO, in effect, becomes the chief educator, tasked with explaining the "why" behind the metric. CMOs must often take a complex message and distill it into a simple format for the team in the trenches to implement. As the leader, it is the CMO's role to ask questions that will help the teams in those trenches build effective processes.

5. Compliance with regulatory agencies

CMOs help hospitals to maintain their conditions of participation (CoP) with the Centers for Medicare and Medicaid Services (CMS). As noted previously, CMS recognizes certain "deemed organizations," as having the capability and authority to verify that hospitals meet the CoP. In many cases, the deemed organization is the Joint Commission, an independent, tax-exempt 501(c)(3) organization that accredits more than twenty-two thousand US health care organizations and programs. The Joint Commission visits hospitals every three years to do a survey.

Other deemed organizations include state regulators. They survey hospitals on a regular triennial schedule or as needed, maybe due to a complaint by a patient, an associate, or someone else. The deemed organization can come in at any point and do an audit, which means they can go anywhere in the hospital. They're like a special counsel; they have superpowers and can review any department in the hospital. If they find something impermissible, they can cite the organization for any number of infractions. Various levels of citations exist, including immediate jeopardy (IJ). Facilities have seven days to respond to an IJ; if they fail to do so, they can be shut down. One such example happened recently in Chicago. CMS closed a hospital because it did not meet the CoP. It's a big deal.

It's the responsibility of the CMO, along with other team members, to make sure that the hospital maintains its CoP. If CMS prohibits a hospital from accepting more CMS patients, it can significantly affect the hospital's financial stability.

One CMS regulation states that no patient can die in a restraint—and multiple definitions of "restraint" exist. A restraint could be mittens, or a physical restraint on the wrist, or an enclosure bed (something like a crib). A patient dying while in restraint is described as a "sentinel event," which must be reported to the state.

Another hospital where I worked many years ago received an immediate jeopardy notice after a patient in a behavioral health unit died in a restraint. We had seven days to create and submit a response (and not seven business days). We all worked through the weekend, then submitted our sixteen-page response, which was accepted. Representatives from the deemed organization visited the hospital and validated our response, and the IJ was removed. Another example of hospitals working to comply with government regulations is the mandatory time-out procedure before surgical operations. This procedure involves marking the surgical site, ensuring all equipment is ready, and confirming the surgical plan with the whole surgical team. Many compare this time-out procedure to aviation checklists, where pilots and other airline personnel habitually and religiously work through long lists of procedures to prevent errors and to ensure that an aircraft is safe to fly. In hospitals, the CMO is crucial to ensuring compliance with the time-out procedure.

Complying with regulations does more than keep a hospital out of trouble. It is this continuous quality assurance, coupled with quality improvement, that keeps the hospital doors open and provides safe patient care. The CMO is key to the success of any survey.

6. Growth, especially with new service lines

Hospitals in growth mode typically look for new service lines to add to their existing services. They must ask, "What is the right service line that we can safely provide on our campus? And what do we need to do to provide that safely?"

CMOs play a leading role in these discussions. First, as previously noted, we need to make sure we have the right process, people, and equipment in place. All three must be ready *before* we start a new service line.

It's incumbent upon a CMO to ensure that the hospital does a failure mode and effects analysis (FMEA) before starting a new service line. An FMEA requires that the hospital's leadership clearly and comprehensively think through the entire service line, gather all the affected team members, and carefully walk through the entire scenario. This team, led by the CMO, should identify potential barriers, consider possible negative outcomes, and discuss solutions to successfully implement the new services.

The team must ask itself, "Do we have the right equipment? Is the CT equipment we already have adequate for the new service? How will handoffs take place? How will the OR team take this equipment to the ICU? What kind of monitor do we have in the ICU? Physicians, do you have the right protocols?" and so on. *All* of that must be done before the launch of a new service.

If a hospital plans to expand or close certain lines, it must inform the state. Trauma and stroke regulations vary by state, with each assigning its own trauma and stroke levels. A hospital must notify the state and obtain approval before adding a cardiac catheterization capability, for example. State representatives will visit your campus to evaluate the facility for compliance with all state and CMS criteria. The hospital must await state clearance before initiating patient care. State inspectors may include doctors, nurses, infection preventionists, and nonclinical facilities experts. Those are generally the four categories of individuals who will make up the state's inspection team.

A CMO will certainly be a crucial part of any team contemplating a hospital's new service line and more than likely will be asked to lead that team. To do so effectively requires the CMO to have an adequate knowledge base, to be able to lead disparate personalities through stressful situations, to be ready to ask difficult and sometimes thorny questions, and to have a very good idea of how much the service line will cost to set up and operate, as well as what kind of income it is likely to generate once operational. It's quite a challenge, but gifted CMOs relish every moment of it!

Hospitals Need CMOs

The strong leadership of a motivated CMO can spell the difference between a thriving hospital and one that's just barely surviving. Successful CMOs know that interdepartmental and interdisciplinary collaboration leads to improved patient safety, better quality, and enhanced hospital performance overall.

Without question, *all* hospitals need an energetic, people-friendly, highly qualified chief medical officer. Their leadership is essential for the hospital's success and sustainability. And in the years to come, the need will only grow more acute.

PART 3

Characteristics of an Effective CMO

How can you excel as a chief medical officer? As mentioned in prior chapters, much of your success will depend on increasing your emotional intelligence. Fortunately, that is an acquired competency we will explore further in this final part.

Certain skills will come in handy as you lead multidisciplinary meetings with physicians and other health care team members. How do you connect with such a diverse group and get their buy-in? Running effective meetings requires good time management, clear information sharing, and actionable plans.

Finally, team-building skills and leading with influence are at the core of being an effective CMO. In part 3, we will examine all these subjects in greater detail.

7

SUPERB PEOPLE INTERACTION

What qualities enable someone to become an effective CMO? Allen Verrill, an MD who now serves as the CEO of a large health care organization, sees humility, curiosity, and a burning desire to communicate as many times and in as many ways as needed as essential qualities. But he doesn't stop there:

> I also think CMOs need to have the patience to know that everything is a process. We as physicians are trained to go straight at something and then think that it's done. Business and operational aspects of hospitals or health care involve far more uncertainty than clinical medicine. If you need to influence many people, you must clearly and repeatedly communicate your goals to guide their actions.
>
> Although in the clinical realm, we learn quite well as the masters of our domain, we're not very good on the business side of medicine. We think everything should be easy, and it's not. That constant reiteration and communication is key. You must be willing to go back into the conversation because you're not being effective, or at least you're not being effective enough to get to where the organization needs to go.

Elise MacCarroll-Wright, a hospital CEO in Illinois, declared that "some of the best CMOs I have worked with have the ability to look beyond just the medical staff goals and how they can align the medical staff goals with the organizational strategy and goals. So, if the organization wants to grow, improve quality, and improve financial sustainability, a good CMO understands how to better align the medical staff with those goals and is able to use their clinical credibility, their partnership, their communication skills, and their influence to get the medical staff to move in that direction. They have to be able to de-escalate complex confrontations. They must be able to collaborate with other C-suite members like CEOs, CFOs, and CIOs. They have to be able to build trust, not just with employed physicians but with independent physicians. They need a lot of people skills and must be oriented toward creating and building partnerships."

Much of what Verrill and MacCarroll-Wright describe depends on developing good relationships. In my view, four key qualities go a long way toward making an effective CMO:

- high emotional intelligence (EQ),
- empathy,
- integrity, and
- the ability to lead through relationships.

Let's take a deeper dive into each of these qualities.

High Emotional Intelligence (EQ)

Training in medicine does not prepare most physicians to lead as a CMO. Clinical excellence does not automatically equate to excellent leadership. Physicians are taught to be strong, to make quick decisions, and to compartmentalize their emotions. They have little time to build strong relationships, which works against achieving high emotional intelligence. Fortunately, EQ is a learned skill set—and if you want to be an effective CMO, you must prioritize that pursuit.

Psychologist Daniel Goleman ignited a helpful revolution in 1995 when he published his runaway bestseller, *Emotional Intelligence: Why*

It Can Matter More Than IQ. Emotional intelligence is the ability to recognize, understand, and manage your own emotions while also recognizing, understanding, and influencing the emotions of others, and then using this new awareness to guide your thinking and behavior. It has five components: *self-awareness*, *self-regulation*, *motivation*, *empathy*, and *social skills*.

While IQ is fixed, EQ can be increased through both learning and practice. In thirty years of studying EQ, researchers have determined that while IQ accounts for only 20 percent of life success, the other 80 percent comes from other factors, including EQ.

When I began my leadership journey, I noticed many opportunities to increase my own EQ. I discovered, for example, that believing I knew everything made me less patient with process changes. Physicians new to leadership find that improving their EQ is especially challenging. Consider a situation in which a physician with newly appointed leadership responsibilities is asked to lead a team of specialists tohaseach a consensus for a process change that has been in existence for a long time. That's no easy task! *Everyone* in the group is a peer, has mastered their art, and has practiced in a certain way for many years. Their training demands quick thinking, a quick response to a crisis, and the right answers. There's no time for a debate during a code blue! Everyone follows the leader—the physician. We spend over twenty thousand hours learning and working in medicine's hierarchical system. The kind of leadership required for the CMO role demands that we let go of our old habits, learn to work in a different environment, and develop a new skill set.

As you might expect, early in my career as a CMO, I ran headlong into several brick walls, leading to many insightful character-strengthening events. Once, I was asked to lead a quality improvement project, and as I customarily did, I approached it already "knowing" the answer. Anyone who launches into a project with that mindset will quickly find themselves butting heads with team members. And then what happens? You get upset that they're not taking your solution! How *dare* they? *You* are the leader.

It didn't take long for me to recognize that I had to scale back my attitude. And while that was a start, it was not nearly enough. I quickly realized that I needed a different strategy. This is self-awareness. We have to realize what needs to change in our approach to get better. The second trigger that prompted me to intentionally work on this skill set is a core requirement for *any* leadership role: the ability to hold effective, crucial conversations. Individuals who have difficulty understanding different perspectives tend to approach conversations with confidence in their own views and therefore try to foist them upon everyone else.

Remember, EQ is a learned skill that comes with time. After each conversation, reflect on what you could do differently next time. If you want to be an effective CMO, focus on growing your emotional intelligence. Make it your priority. Learn that skill and then continually get better at it through practice.

Another important aspect of this skill is the ability to receive feedback. Physicians take pride in their work, which often leads to taking things personally. We must shift our mindset. Do not interpret all feedback as personal criticism.

Former CEO Ken Lukhard told me, "I had a few CMOs early on in my career who weren't that great. I had to fire one because he was just so self-centered, so arrogant. I had to fire him, although he'd been there a long time. I was a young CEO, but it was worth that bloody battle because I knew that so long as he was in that chair, the hospital could not flourish. I have encountered some individuals who faced challenges in this area and did not remain, but those whom I selected or mentored contributed significantly to the organization. They have a skill set that I don't have and that nobody else in the C-suite has, and thus the importance of their role."

Ken also recognized the crucial role of EQ in the skill set of a CMO:

> In my mind, you're looking for a rare combination of talents in a chief medical officer. Among them is what I would call a high EQ. You want people who have a very strong sense of emotional intelligence. That's both internal and external, in terms of their ability to monitor not only what's going on inside of them but also what's going on in the room around them. Those are the kind of people I looked for in hiring CMOs.

Empathy

Although empathy is officially considered a part of EQ, I think it's valuable to consider it on its own. Empathy, too, is a learned skill. Although some individuals are born with more empathy than others, anyone can learn it through their own life experiences, whether personal or professional. Empathy is crucial when dealing with hospitalized patients who are in the most vulnerable time of their lives. We need compassionate leaders standing beside them.

In a CMO role, empathy translates to trying to understand the other person's perspective. Understanding my physicians' perspectives helps me become a better leader. But that can happen *only* if I invest in the critical learned skill of active listening. We become more empathetic by practicing active listening.

Active listening requires us to concentrate, understand, respond appropriately, and then remember what has been said. It demands that we improve our attention span and lean into a conversation. Unfortunately, the medical training of physicians makes this highly unnatural for most of us.

A 2017 study published in *JAMA* referenced two previous studies, one conducted in 1984 and the second in 1999. They both explored how frequently clinicians asked their patients about their main concerns *and* how long they listened to their patients' stories before interrupting them. These studies, performed fifteen years apart, found that patients given the opportunity to tell their story tended to be quickly interrupted. But the most striking finding of these studies was not the nature or ultimate effect of the interruptions, but the fact that after asking patients to express their concerns, physicians listened to their patients' stories for a median of only *eighteen-to-twenty-three seconds* before interrupting.[131]

Another study in the *Journal of General Internal Medicine* found that physicians interrupted patients after a median of only *eleven* seconds. The study reported that "patients who were not interrupted only spoke for a median of six seconds. Our opinion is this suggests more about physician patience (and as suggested by Drs. Mohammed and Yueng, time constraints) than about the time required for patients to relay their agenda and story. Many patients who spoke only briefly had no concerns and thus had minimal opportunity for interruption. If they in fact did have a concern or more prolonged story behind their chief complaint, they were interrupted only a few seconds into their story."[132]

Now, don't get me wrong. Sometimes, interruptions can help guide a clinical encounter. And yet the article concludes, "we continue to purport that seconds into the initial elicitation of the patient's concerns is not the appropriate time for interjection."[133] Indeed, such a pivotal part of the medical encounter should allow the patient to relay their story and, in return, experience their physician's engaged, empathetic listening rather than a quick question and answer–driven conversation. "More importantly," the article said, "the main finding of our study is that the time to interruption of the patient's agenda continues to be measured in seconds."[134] On average, that's how quickly we stop listening to patients.

I challenge you to try an experiment. How long do you wait before interrupting? I was in denial until I clocked my own seconds. The experiment is an eye-opener.

A related technique that I had to intentionally lean into was learning *listen to learn*, not *listen to respond*. This is the basis of active listening. When you are in a conversation, your mind should pause and not move on to building a response or preparing your next question. That is only "hearing." We need to pause, lean in, and "listen." Active listening means putting down the cell phone or pager and working to understand the message. We should begin our response only after asking any necessary follow-up questions. There's a big difference between hearing and listening.

In certain respects, our medical training has influenced us to conceal expressions of empathy. We move from one patient's room to the next, addressing both our responsibilities and the patients' needs. Some days, we move rapidly from handling a death to delivering a new life next door. We are trained to compartmentalize our emotions so that we can quickly take care of a different patient suffering from another problem. It's ingrained in us. Even if by nature we have empathy, our training teaches us to hide it or squelch it. When we become physician leaders, we must unlearn everything we were taught about empathy. We must instead approach empathy as an indispensable learned skill.

For me, the transformation began to take place during a critical coaching moment. One day, my executive coach taught me what he called "the five-second pause." As a young CMO, I grew very anxious whenever I lacked an immediate response to some question. I thought I needed to know everything. Today, I understand that I don't know everything and that I don't *need* to know everything. I don't have to give an immediate reply to someone's question; I can pause for five seconds. I've also learned to say, "I don't have the answer right now. May I get back to you on it?"

Many young CMOs don't realize they *can* pause for five seconds. It may sound easy to do, but believe me, it's *very* difficult at first! The room goes quiet as everyone waits for your response. You need to grow comfortable with that pause.

Empathetic leadership is a deliberate choice. It won't just happen. This part of the journey requires deliberate effort.

CMOs must express empathy not only toward patients but also toward their physician colleagues. Physician burnout is no myth, and we live in a cultural moment when physician suicides have skyrocketed (see chapter 4). As leaders, CMOs must be aware of that grim reality. An empathetic CMO will lean in, spot a distressed colleague, and have a thoughtful conversation. Peer-to-peer support is the strongest tactic we can utilize to help physicians better cope with stress.

One director of risk at a midwestern hospital told me, "It's important for CMOs to listen. The CMO should listen to the risk manager's scenario without becoming defensive. They must remain receptive to information from different perspectives and be ready to respond, including engaging in discussions with the provider. That doesn't necessarily mean having to share the follow-up specific to that conversation, because that might be confidential. But the team will have the sense that their concern is taken seriously. If the provider's behavior changes, we know that action was taken. It's very important to listen without getting defensive."

Empathy is shown through the spontaneous recognition of physician-led problem-solving. When doctors know that the CMO appreciates their hard work, morale improves. It's all part of learning and practicing the skill of empathy.

Integrity

Integrity is a critical trait for every CMO; it's also one of the high reliability pillars (see chapter 9). I define integrity as doing the right thing all the time, every time, because it's the right thing to do, not because somebody is watching. Consistently acting with integrity builds trust, which is essential in working effectively with physicians.

For a physician in the trenches, integrity may translate into doing a time-out in the OR because it's the right thing to do, not because somebody is watching. For a CMO having contract conversations with physicians, integrity demands that the CMO put energy and considerable thought into those negotiations. They should also make the effort to close the feedback loop. Physicians want to hear from the CMO about developments in many areas; they don't ever want to feel shut out of critical conversations that affect them. Closing the feedback loop helps to build trust, which requires doing the right thing because it is the right thing to do.

Any time a physician asks me a question, I try to give them an update as quickly as possible, even if the update is only, "I have not forgotten about you; it is still in the works." I've found they appreciate that. If I don't do that, I break the trust loop, which reveals poor integrity.

During an executive search for the position of medical director, I helped explore the role with an interested physician. Three weeks later, I realized I had not circled back, so I sent her an email saying, "Don't think that I've forgotten. Conversations are still happening in the back end. We will set up a one-on-one very soon."

Within a day, I received a note from her. "I so appreciate this email," she said.

That's what physicians want. They don't necessarily want a final answer; they want to be kept in the loop and be updated regularly.

A CMO's integrity means earning trust from all peers. If I don't do the right thing all the time, the CEO, to whom I report, will lose trust in me. I must "manage up" my supervisors. What strategies can I employ to effectively manage upward when I sense a lack of trust from my manager? Trust will grow only if I do the right thing all the time. If I make a mistake, I admit it and keep everyone informed.

The same process must occur at every level. My dyad partner is the chief nursing officer. If they don't see me doing the right thing, or if they see me wavering, I will never generate trust with my nursing colleagues, the largest workforce in a hospital that directly impacts patient care. A CMO cannot function without building trust, which requires behaving with integrity with *all* peers. Integrity requires managing up, down, and sideways.

Dr. Rick Scott, one of my mentors, was always honest with me and kept me in the loop. I had a very different experience with another CMO who habitually gave me only partial information. She was young and in her first gig as a CMO. No doubt she later became an entirely different leader, but at the time, I found it difficult to trust her. Keeping everyone informed builds trust, which underpins integrity.

Dr. Scott described another incident for me in which a lack of integrity led to serious consequences:

> I think of a rare instance when a medical staff had to be prompted into restricting or removing privileges from a well-connected staff member whose practice was no longer meeting community or professional standards. The surgeon in question was also the "most productive" member of his department.
>
> Medical staff become like small communities (or dysfunctional families) and often are loath to negatively impact someone whose children are in school with theirs, or perhaps whose spouses are friends. Maybe they relied on them in consultation for patient care in the past. But people change over time, skills don't keep up, and financial pressures may cloud judgment.
>
> My site CMO felt reluctant to make a call to action, even when quality issues became clear. His boss wondered where the case volume would go if the surgeon were removed—but *not* whether the cases themselves were appropriate. Quality reviews and fair hearing processes are unhappy events, but they're often necessary. It's the CMO who must be the unwavering conscience of the medical staff.

Rick summed up his story like this: "The CMO is the careful gardener, and sometimes, things need pruning for the garden to thrive."

For Alan Kaplan, a longtime physician and the CEO of University of Wisconsin Health, behaving with integrity means being "consistent and respectful, and communicating proactively. If I'm approachable and demonstrate integrity that goes beyond honesty, then my physician credibility helps. But if I don't exhibit those things, then it doesn't matter. You still have to be a good leader."[135]

The Ability to Lead Through Relationships

Why do we so highly value EQ and empathy? Why do we insist on integrity? A CMO does so for one primary reason: Better relationships among hospital staff lead to better outcomes for our patients. A white paper from the American Association for Physician Leadership declared:

> Physicians . . . must work with professional clinical teams in a complex environment. Without exception, thought leaders in the field of physician leadership emphasize the critical requirement of building great teams and working with them effectively. But they also point out how challenging it can be for physicians to transition from the independent thinking driven into them in medical training programs to the interdependence of working with a team.
>
> Although many physicians tend toward autonomy and independence, it is important to recognize that this behavior can directly or indirectly impede successful patient care outcomes. It also can create barriers to forming, leading, or participating in successful teams.[136]

The author concluded that "physicians must develop deeper insights into why they resist working on teams and learn how they can modulate and channel this behavior into positive action without losing their pride and passion."[137] That advice goes double for CMOs.

One experienced hospital CFO told me,

> A good CMO understands the prevailing campus climate by nurturing good relationships with the clinicians. What most concerns them? What do they want? What's the end goal? Some want to grow their practice or perhaps bring in a partner so they can retire. A good CMO gets the backstory on these issues by developing healthy relationships with everyone involved.
>
> Even in physician leadership meetings, the CMO speaks with physicians to understand their issues. Are they having difficulty getting a patient into the OR? Are they having trouble getting a schedule? Do they wonder how the GI recovery space is going? Do they worry about how patient follow-up is not happening? The CMO brings all of that back to our executive meetings, but not in an accusatory way. She'll say, "Here's the feedback I'm getting from physicians. The recovery area is not conducive to the physician. The staffing's not right, and they're not feeling comfortable."

A CMO acts as the sounding board for *all* such concerns. "I value CMOs who do that," the CFO continued. "They have a unique set of knowledge, and they bring it to the table whenever we sit down to negotiate, or even when we have a conversation about expanding a service. They have those conversations *way* before bringing the issue to a committee for a vote. We come to understand the passion of our physicians and why they want something. Great CMOs do that back work all the time."

One chief nursing officer declared that, from a safety and quality perspective, a CMO and CNO "must have a very tight relationship. The CMO keeps me apprised of developments in medicine. I sit on the medical executive committee, along with the chairs of the other departments. I get to hear what concerns them. I get to hear if nursing played a role in some incident or if physicians did. I am the only nurse who sits on that committee."

The CNO's predecessor was essentially seen but not heard on that committee. "The CMO changed that up for me," she said. "Now, the president of the medical staff will often ask for my perspective on some issue. The CMO helped me build a strong relationship with the physicians."

Unfortunately, that had not always been true. During her first year, the CNO was employed at a community hospital that had no obstetrical peer review process in place. Any time a medical physician problem arose in the obstetrical gynecology area, it went to the hospital peer review, which the CNO thought was "kind of funny, because there was no OB/GYN sitting on that peer review. I'm not quite sure how they did a peer review. It took me a whole year of working with the chair of OB/GYN to persuade the previous CMO to even get that committee going. That CMO was not very supportive. When a new CMO arrived, she backed my idea and joined the committee as my dyad. Before then, I was unable, as a nurse, to tell the chairman of the department how peer review works. I tried to explain, but it never clicked with them. Once the new CMO started attending those meetings, she guided the chair of the department and the other OB/GYNs sitting on that committee about how to deal with a bad outcome. That was one big area that she was able to help me with."

Treating your colleagues with respect is not only the right thing to do, but it also pays big dividends. "I value the respect and courtesy I get from my CMO," this CNO said. "We respect each other's roles. A former CNO would say to the CMO, 'This is nursing. You stay in your lane, and I'll stay in my lane.' We've never done that. *Ever*. We respect each other too much to create artificial lanes. Sometimes she will say to me, 'No, I don't think that's right. What do you think?' I present my perspective to her directly, and she responds by saying, 'I understand your point of view.' She extends the same courtesy to me when sharing her own thoughts."[138]

That's true dyad leadership. There is enough evidence in medical literature to support this style of leadership. I've worked to model it and hardwire it in every unit of our hospitals.

A 2024 MDA Leadership white paper characterizes the dyad leadership model in health care as a partnership between a physician leader and an administrator who jointly provide strategic and operational oversight. This model has been adopted by 77 percent of health care organizations globally, with 85 percent believing it is effective. The model is particularly beneficial in health care environments where the need for high-quality leadership is paramount. It allows for the integration of clinical expertise with business acumen, leading to improved patient care and operational efficiency. The model has been in use since 1908 at the Mayo Clinic and continues to be a key component of effective health care leadership.[139]

One hospital's director of quality and patient safety spoke of the necessity of having what she called "an active relationship" between the quality and patient safety team and the CMO, primarily to ensure continuous support and collaboration. She sees this relationship as crucial for ensuring excellent quality, patient safety, and regulatory compliance.

"It's also important to emphasize collaboration and open dialogue in decision-making," she said. "I think a good CMO allows for differing opinions and values the expertise of others, which leads to better outcomes for patient safety and quality. It's crucial to build trust and good working relationships, which are essential within the health care team. Removing hierarchical barriers makes more effective communication and collaboration possible, which also leads to better patient safety and quality outcomes."[140]

Physician Well-Being

Physician well-being is a huge part of developing healthy relationships in any organization (see chapter 4). CMOs must be champions of physician well-being, as no one understands the stresses of physicians as much as the CMOs who have walked in their shoes. We therefore must support our physicians through a strong focus on well-being, especially after an adverse event.

Physicians and nursing teams often become second victims of traumatic events. Surgeons, especially, tend to be very reticent to share their feelings, preferring to hide behind a stoic demeanor (a natural result of their training). As already noted, most of us learned to compartmentalize our emotions during residency training. The fast pace meant we were constantly faced with life and death on the same day. We were taught that we must never linger on the sad; we must move on to the neutral (if not happy) place.

These days, thankfully, the situation is slowly but steadily changing. Today, after a death in a code, young physicians in training are taught to pause, gather around the patient, and if the patient's family is present, pray with them with or without the chaplain. This supports healing not only for the patient's family but also the staff and physicians themselves.

My initial experience with this happened a few years after completing my residency. As the hospitalist on duty, I needed to hold a compassionate discussion with a family about a terminal ventilator withdrawal. After the patient had passed and the family was gathered, the chaplain on duty called an impromptu prayer in the room. I was caught off guard as the chaplain extended her hand toward me, and we all gathered as a small group as she led the prayer. I am certain it provided comfort for the family. I also felt a great peace descend on *me*. The passing of a soul and the deep humanness of the situation were palpable at that very moment. I will forever remember that day.

If physicians are not emotionally well and have begun to show signs of burnout, it impacts all of us, including our patients. The CMO is responsible for overseeing the health and well-being of *all* colleagues. We must keep an eye out for one another by having each other's backs.

"Whenever we're in front of our physicians or nursing colleagues," said one experienced CNO about her relationship with her CMO, "what matters most is trust. Of all the people I've ever worked with, my CMO has my back, 110 percent. She may provide feedback privately on how situations could be improved, but publicly, we support each other. We are a united force. We build trust by laying out what we need to do prior to doing it. I mean, we have a meeting before the meeting. She points out possible failures, and I explain actions and potential nursing-related risks. We go in as a united force. We both feel that quality is our number one priority, so we trust each other. She helps me understand a physician's thinking, and I help her understand a nurse's thought process."

Because I have my colleagues' backs and earnestly desire their well-being, I will not text my colleagues after hours about work unless it is an emergency. I don't want them to feel compelled to respond. If I do text or email them, I add a disclaimer at the end.

I firmly believe it is the duty of every CMO to help decrease burnout among medical staff and build resilience. While physicians in general are a resilient force by the sheer nature of their work, some studies claim that an average of *one physician every day* commits suicide. Obviously, something is awry here.

As practicing physicians, our personal and professional well-being depends squarely on what we do and how we react. I view this as an important CMO responsibility, and I therefore approach it with care. All clinicians need to be mindful of each other's well-being, or else their own well-being might become collateral damage.

A Sacred Task

All of us start our careers with the idealism and energy of youth. We believe that we can change the world. We enter this noble profession to positively impact the lives of our fellow human beings.

Each generation views medicine in its own way. Baby boomers likely will have a harder time acclimating to digital medicine than millennials or Gen Zers. These days, children hold an iPad before they can hold a pen! Such changes often lead to different types and layers of frustration.

Remember that the only thing we can influence is how we react. We can let cynicism become our universe, or we can focus on what we can impact. We can determine to help each other successfully journey through the unique world of medicine. And guess what? My well-being depends on my colleague's emotional stability, and vice versa. We cannot effectively address burnout in isolation. We must seek help and listen to each other, removing in the process the stigma attached to reaching out. This is a sign of strength, not of weakness.

Merriam-Webster defines well-being as "the state of being happy, healthy, or prosperous."[141] Sounds so simple, doesn't it? Then why is it so difficult to achieve? Is it due to competing priorities or to the constant want of something more? I think of an old saying here: "Be thankful, as your life could be someone else's fairy tale."

We may choose to focus on the thorn or the rose, or to generate negative or positive energy. We choose how we react. We can choose to say thank you or sorry and mean it. Those are two of the most powerful statements we can make to impact the person across the room.

Be well and be happy. It is not difficult—but it does take conscious, intentional effort. Do it for yourself and for your colleagues, because we don't want well-being to become our collateral damage. We are a smart group; I am certain we can figure it out.

8

EXTENSIVE LIFE EXPERIENCE

Why don't good CMO candidates just stride onto the scene right out of medical school? Why can't you take a course titled CMO 101 and immediately qualify for the position? The reason is simple. Regardless of someone's intelligence, passions, interests, and academic training, it takes a good chunk of life experience and willingness to serve well as a chief medical officer.

In this chapter, I'd like to highlight four key elements of life experience that every effective CMO must have:

- successful clinical experience,
- proven leadership skills, especially in team building,
- a willingness to self-invest, and
- proficiency in time management.

Successful Clinical Experience

To succeed in their position, CMOs need credibility among their peers—and the only way to get such credibility is to have a clear record of successful clinical experience. No CMO can gain the necessary respect of their medical colleagues without it. It simply won't happen.

How much clinical experience is needed? I believe that any CMO candidate needs at least ten to fifteen years of fruitful clinical experience before they're ready for the unique demands of the position. It can be any kind of clinical experience—internal medicine, pediatrics, surgery, neurology, ER, OB/GYN, you name it—but you must be a practicing physician who has metaphorically walked in the shoes of your physician colleagues. You must be able to understand the stresses, challenges, and pain they're going through. You must also have a knack for translating all of that in the administrative corridors to help your colleagues deliver the care they're tasked with providing. This can happen *only* with a significant amount of real-life experience. I cannot emphasize it enough: A successful CMO must have extensive and fruitful clinical experience. It's a nonnegotiable. Physicians will respect their clinical administrative lead only if he or she has clinical credibility in their eyes.

"We don't respect a physician who can't practice good clinical medicine," said Allen Verrill, MD, the president and CEO of Advent-Health Shawnee Mission. "I think it's a core criterion that you must have been a good physician at some level, to some degree, for at least several years before you can step into the leadership realm. You need to have done the work and done it well to gain the respect of those around you. Otherwise, it devalues the practice of what we do in the fraternity and sorority of medicine. I think most physicians can identify those who did it well versus those who didn't, even if they've never seen the person practice. Reputationally, they'll seek it out. They'll ask about the individual and investigate. It's hard to be a good CMO if you don't have clinical expertise and the reputation of having practiced well. The credibility that comes with experience is a core criterion for the position, but that does *not* qualify someone to be an outstanding CMO. It's just the minimum criteria."

According to Peter B. Angood, MD, writing in a white paper published by the American Association for Physician Leadership, "A shared history and a common language give physician leaders the credibility among their colleagues and other providers needed to garner critical support for clinical integration. This support allows them to drive the value agenda for initiatives such as reducing variations in care, reducing readmissions, developing a patient-centered medical home, implementing best practices, and other value-driven strategies."[142]

Physicians are curious by nature and in a lifelong learning mode. We earn CMEs, we obtain certifications for new procedures, we show competency every reappointment cycle, we give lectures and maintain certification in various fields of medicine, and we do all of this with pride. We invest in ourselves clinically.

When we step into the unknown territory of administrative medicine, we must approach it with the same kind of rigor. To build credibility, we must invest in our own administrative learning. We change hats and take leadership courses, earn administrative certifications, choose lifelong learning in a new field of medicine, and learn to play in a square toolbox rather than from the top of a hierarchical pyramid. All of this takes practice and intentionality. But in the end, it all helps build credibility in the eyes of our colleagues and peers.

Exactly as with other C-suite leadership roles, the CMO position is an administrative-only position. An outdated myth persists in some circles that a CMO can do both clinical and administrative work. Such a dual function can no longer work. The demands of the position are much more extensive and complex than in years past, which makes it impossible to remain competent in both worlds at the same time. *No* contemporary full-time CMO can split time between administrative and clinical duties. One task must go.

A July 2025 article in *Becker's Clinical Leadership* touted the idea of splitting leadership roles as part administrative, part clinical, but this practice works best in academic medicine. Research, teaching, mentoring, training, clinical trials, data review, policy recommendation, problem-solving for specific issues—all these activities can be successfully pursued with a willing physician splitting time between clinical and administrative duties or in non-CMO roles only.

"Departments create their own roles and structure for split time depending on their needs," the article explained. "Some physicians may only spend 5% of their time on administrative or teaching duties, while others might spend 90%. Across academic medical centers, the most common division appears to be 20% to 25% spent on administrative or faculty roles."[143]

Don't miss the phrase "across academic medical centers"! Such a strategy cannot work for a contemporary CMO working in a nonacademic health care setting. And why should it? We do not expect the CFO of a hospital to run another business, do we? Or do we require a CNO to practice at a patient's bedside? Why, then, would anyone expect a CMO to juggle clinical and administrative duties?

It is critical that a health care organization's key clinical leadership remains laser focused on the organizational key quality indicators, and the only way to do this is to fully commit to the administrative component.

Leadership Skills and Team Building

All physicians are leaders in the clinical setting. They are trained to focus on their patients one person at a time, to lead a code with confidence and knowledge, and to be competitive.

How can a physician leader manage a team in an environment that emphasizes active listening, encourages input from all members, and requires the leader to reserve their own perspective until others have shared theirs, even if they believe they already have a solution? Such leadership does not come naturally to most physicians. Physicians are *not* traditional leaders. It is a skill set that must be acquired. We can *become* good leaders.

To acquire this skill set, we need some basic leadership knowledge first. One good way to acquire it is by attending leadership institute courses (*before* taking the CMO job). Think of this as your leadership foundation. Once you have that solid, core foundation in place, the additional leadership lessons you learn through experience can move you steadily forward.

As a seasoned CMO, I've mentored more than one physician who was hoping and preparing to one day become a CMO or even a regional CMO. One promising young physician, two years into a

CMO role, was given an opportunity to excel . . . and she declined it. I wanted to know why. "Why did you say no to that?" I asked her. "*You* are my succession plan. A few years from now, I'm going to retire. Why did you give up this opportunity to show the leadership that you are the right person for the job?" I asked open-ended questions so that I could understand her mindset. Did she have the required understanding? Did she have a higher comprehension of her own role?

Through our conversation, I grasped that she felt bogged down in non-CMO duties. On further exploration, I discovered that she was leading efforts that were clearly the responsibility of the CEO or the CNO. I encouraged her to have some difficult conversations with her administrative colleagues and offload some of those duties to create space on her plate to spend time on quality and patient safety—the sole responsibilities of a CMO.

As her leader and her battle buddy, I realized that it was up to me to build her up and give her the knowledge she needed to succeed. I believe it's the responsibility of every leader and executive to work on their own succession plan. Effective leadership ensures successful transitions by making processes systematic rather than reliant on individuals. That is true legacy.

CMOs must interact and collaborate with their operational leaders to impact all kinds of critical areas, including but not limited to length of stay, the case mix index (CMI), operating room efficiency, and throughput. CMOs cannot do this alone; they must partner with care management leaders to impact LOS, with clinical documentation leaders to impact CMI, with OR leaders to improve first case on time starts (FCOTs), and with the COO to impact throughput. All of these are key metrics that make up the lifeline of any hospital operation.

Ken Lukhard, who until his retirement served for thirty years as the president/CEO of medical centers and regional health care markets, is also a recipient of the American College of Healthcare Executives's Lifetime Achievement Award. He says about finding excellent CMO candidates, "My experience tells me that you look for people who are smart and show a natural aptitude to lead. They have good leadership qualities innately. People tend to follow them. They're good leaders, they're good listeners, they know how to build teams, and they know how to ask questions. They're not autocratic knuckleheads."

Team-Building Skills

Although the ability to build teams is crucial for all health care organizations, most physicians don't know how to do it well. I admit that team building was the most difficult skill that I had to learn. But once again, it's a *learned* skill.

Why is this so difficult for physicians? In their clinical training, physicians spend twenty thousand hours with people who constantly tell them, "*You* are the leader. *You're* going to call the shots, whether you're performing surgery in the operating room or running a code blue on the floors. You *don't* call for a teammate. You *don't* look around and ask for information. The buck stops with *you*."

I speak from experience. Five panicked seconds of my life have continued to stay with me for decades.

I was fresh out of residency. I wasn't a naive resident or unfamiliar with the practice of medicine. I was a mature resident, a graduate of two residency programs.

Nurses get twelve weeks of orientation and a buddy system once they start working in a hospital, but no similar onboarding exists for a physician. Physicians are just let loose in a new ICU or an OR and are basically told, "Go figure it out. Manage and use this equipment that you've never used before. Take care of a patient by yourself," although until then, they've always had an attending physician looking over their shoulder.

When I walked into an ICU for the very first time, fresh out of my second residency, a nurse speaking to someone on the phone looked at me and said, "Don't worry, the attending just walked in." I glanced around to see who she meant. And then it occurred to me: *Oh, that's me!* Despite my panic, my training kicked in within five seconds, and

I took over. I didn't have time to build a team or build rapport with the staff. I took care of the patient and managed the needs of this sick person in the ICU.

I tell this story repeatedly because team-building skills are not part of a physician's medical training. All CMOs must *learn* how to build teams. While a physician typically thinks only about their patient, as the CMO, I must slow down and think about the perspectives of other team members. Those who serve in the CMO role must think about a whole community, not merely a single individual.

I recently spoke to an OB doctor who works in the emergency department. "We have six parking spaces in front of my OB/ED," she told me. "I would like you to mark all of them, 'Restricted to OB/ED positions only.'"

"May I ask, who else uses those spaces?" I replied.

"Oh, general surgeons are always coming in and parking there and taking up our spots," the doc answered. "I want you to restrict that. This is physician well-being! You want us to be engaged? Then do this for me."

That physician was thinking only about her department, which is not wrong. But as the CMO, I must think about *everyone*. "I'll need to talk to the general surgeons," I replied. "I'd like to know why they are parking there."

"They don't have emergencies," she answered.

But how would an OB/ED physician know that? Is it possible that a general surgeon might have a patient who requires emergency abdominal surgery? Or a cardiologist running in for a STEMI? As the CMO, you must constantly think about team building. You must ponder how to build your *team*, which means you must consider the whole house.

In my younger years, I probably would have told the OB/ED doctor, "Sure, this is a low-hanging fruit. I can fix the problem right now," without realizing that my on-the-spot decision might negatively (and even catastrophically) impact a different patient or another physician. That's just basic team building.

Consider another example. How many hospital patients develop a surgical site infection after surgery? Such infections can occur for many reasons. Perhaps the patient wasn't given an antibiotic in a timely fashion, or maybe someone on the surgical team didn't wash their hands. Or perhaps the surgeon changed gloves, or the tray wasn't sterile, or the patient lacked good care at home, or home health workers didn't train the patient on how to properly wash their hands. To help prevent *one* surgical site infection, I'd need to work with *six* teams: the main operating room, the infection prevention team, the providers, the sterile processing department, the floor RNs, and (last but not least) the vendors who deliver the trays for surgeries. That takes extensive team building to avoid a single surgical site infection! I'd need to hardwire these processes and get everybody's buy-in.

Surprisingly, in general, surgeons tend to be the hardest group to convince. I must remind them, "One glove not changed is one patient harmed." When physicians or groups resist change, I must patiently use good data and communicate my rationale in terms they understand.

Not long ago, I had to find a way to convince our surgeons that they needed to change their scrubs before they went into the OR. I showed them the evidence.

"No," they replied. "The pathogens on our scrubs are very different from the pathogens that show up in the infection."

I quickly realized that I needed a team-building exercise, along with a leader among that group to lead the charge. So, I looked for a surgeon who was already practicing this in OR. I spoke to him about the idea. "I'd like you to speak to your own colleagues," I said. "You'll lead this discussion, not me." I asked him to form a coalition of three or four surgeons; I expected the rest to follow. I knew such a strategy would take time (probably months), but we got there.

I deal with patient safety events nearly every day. Every hospital has a system that enables individuals to log their concerns about a process or potential patient harm. Every day, I review these events and follow them with intentionality, whether they require an RCA or are a "near miss." And I ask myself, "What can we do different to positively impact the health of the next patient in a similar clinical scenario?"

Team building must deal effectively with finger-pointing. We must avoid going down unproductive rabbit holes. I often use simple questions to redirect two opposing groups to focus on what's under their control or in their circle of influence. Surely, there must be *something* that they themselves can do differently? This always makes them ponder. Poor processes will fail a competent person every time. Ninety percent of the time, it is the process rather than the individual who is responsible for a potentially poor outcome.

A graphic I saw recently on the web caught my eye. It featured a big circle with a dot in the middle. The big circle was labeled, "This is what the other person is going through," while the dot was labeled, "This is what you know about it." We have no idea why a patient or person behaves as they do. I always return to this idea with my team members. When they come to me complaining, "This was terrible! Just look at this event," I always tell them, "Pause. There are always three sides to a story—yours, the other person's, and the truth. This is one person's perspective. You must listen to the other person before you make a decision."

A CMO needs team-building skills not only when forging alliances between nurses and medical staff, but also when interacting with members of the C-suite. My clinical dyad is the chief nursing officer. Pausing to hear her perspective builds trust and avoids failures that could compromise patient care.

Team-building skills are also extremely important for building rapport with your administrative peers. I try to build rapport with my C-suite peers in several ways. I make time on my calendar for them, or I simply walk into their offices, sit down, and have a chat. I notice family photos on their walls and ask who the people in the photos are. I want us to get to know each other. Showing interest in their lives is *extremely* important. I'll ask, "How's your son doing?" or "What happened at your doctor's appointment?"

Some of my colleagues are young execs with little kids. While I'm not in that boat, I need to be aware and cognizant of those who are. My own executive administrative assistant has young children, whom she drops off every morning. "That's fine," I'll say, "I'll manage. Go drop off your kids. It's important." Or I'll ask, "How was the drop-off?" or "How's soccer going?"

A successful CMO must choose to build those C-suite connections by showing interest in the lives of their administrative colleagues. We are not disembodied heads; we are human beings with full lives apart from medical charts and tight budgets. Successful CMOs remember that.

A Willingness to Self-Invest

Physician leaders who aspire to serve in the CMO role must invest in themselves, something that is very high on my priority list. The willingness to self-invest tells me that a person is eager to learn and zealous in their pursuit of success, and that they have the outlook to do the job well. A willingness to self-invest tells me a great deal about somebody.

While many avenues to invest in yourself exist, I'll focus on just two: advanced degrees beyond the MD/DO and volunteering for roles that can help you explore health care beyond the clinical realm.

Advanced Degrees

If you're thinking about pursuing a CMO role, I highly encourage you to seek an advanced degree outside of clinical medicine. Such a pursuit shows your commitment to enhancing your knowledge base beyond the medical field. Gaining additional education in areas such as business, risk management, or leadership is critical to moving your mindset from being a peer to your colleagues to becoming their clinical leaders. It is a very difficult shift to make! And while not many do it successfully, earning an appropriate advanced degree can help. It's important to earn an MBA, MPH, MHA, or any relevant master's degree (pick one), but you must have that additional degree.

Why? A relevant master's degree broadens the knowledge horizons of a CMO. It helps them better understand the business aspect of medicine, adds to their emotional intelligence, and introduces patient safety through a different lens. I've found it extremely valuable to have that additional degree.

Charles M. Falcone, MD, the director of Korn Ferry, said that when he first started to train as a physician, very few of his colleagues wanted any additional education, let alone to become an executive. Today, however, he says that "a greater number of physicians have advanced business or administrative degrees, like an MBA or MHA. They have chosen to get involved with the decision-making that exists in the C-suite."[144]

In an article titled "Doctors Extending Their Education: *Why an MBA? Is It a Degree of Success?*", Jeffrey B. Kramer, MD, wrote, "What I most enjoyed were two things: looking at the world (including the health care world) from a completely different vantage point and being able to bounce all kinds of ideas off of fellow students and faculty."[145] Kramer then asked, "How can this investment in time be justified?" He answered:

> From my standpoint, physicians need to gain control over the health care system. Unless we can speak the language of business, understand the complexities of health care delivery, and see the health care world from a practical (i.e., business) vantage point, we will be powerless. This is true for employed and independent physicians alike.
>
> Physicians need to be involved. We can sit back and allow events to overtake us, but many of us want to make an impact on the world and make it a better place. If we as individuals don't step up and lead, who will? The MBA gives us tools to get there.

Another MD, Adrian J. Delaney III, declared, "Completing an MBA was my opportunity to understand the anatomy of our health care system . . . I knew that I needed to better myself not only as a physician, but as a leader and a visionary in health care in order to provide the kind of care my patients need and deserve."[146]

Keep this in mind: Self-investing in an additional degree carries much more weight with health care organizations when you voluntarily pay for at least part of that additional education. Rather than saying, "The hospital should send me to this course," or "The system ought to pick up the tuition for my MBA," do it on your own initiative. While many hospitals will chip in for such further education (at least, to some extent), what are *you* doing to self-invest?

When I did my own MBA, the hospital I worked for picked up the cost of tuition for one semester a year; I paid for the rest. When physicians tell me, "You need to pay me to attend this conference," I often respond with a modification of JFK's famous statement: "Ask not what the hospital can do for you—ask what you can do for yourself."

Volunteering for Committee Work

Few people enjoy committee work, but joining key committees in a hospital or health care organization offers valuable insight into how health care operates. Serving on well-chosen committees can prepare you for the duties of a CMO better than almost anything else.

One of my young former physician colleagues has learned this lesson well. He wrote, "To transition into the CMO role, it's essential to move beyond the daily duties of patient care and actively participate in hospital committees. This involvement allows you to find your voice and establish your presence among a team of leaders working together to improve patient outcomes. As your communication and leadership skills grow, you will naturally evolve into a leadership role within the committee, becoming a respected figure whose advice and recommendations are sought after by hospital administration."

Another young colleague, an OB/GYN physician, told me that getting involved in hospital committee work exposed her to the responsibilities of the CMO role and allowed her to see if the role would be a good fit for her. She said, "I attended numerous committee meetings outside my OB/GYN specialty because I was encouraged to observe the daily work of other departments, which broadened my experience beyond what I was clinically trained for. I was still in charge of a lot of quality metrics for the hospital; that's my background. The CMO helped me join several committees to expand my knowledge."[147]

Again, those thinking about pursuing a CMO role need to see this additional work as an investment in themselves. "I think that being constantly proactive and not being scared to do that extra work will help me in my future career," said one young physician. "I believe that if I work hard today, I'll reap the benefits tomorrow. Right now, I have no time carved out for any kind of administrative work; I'm a full-time clinical employee. You face pressure to meet specific metrics. But it's my own time that I'm carving out when I do these extra obligations. I have a vested interest in them. I'm not expecting a monetary return at this point because I'm looking out for my own future. That's how I see it."

Time Management Skills

I've seen repeatedly over my CMO career how critically important time management is. Two skills in this area seem especially important: running meetings and managing your schedule.

Running Meetings

In general, physicians don't like long meetings. They prefer brief sessions with swift decisions and fast results. Those are great—but they don't always happen in a CMO leadership role. Still, whether you're a CMO or a physician in the trenches, one sacred commandment never disappears: *Don't waste my time. If the meeting does not add value to me and I don't add value to the meeting, then it's not a meeting I need to be a part of.*

In general, most physicians learn the skill of running an effective meeting (at least, over time). And once they learn it, they don't forget it. Every CMO needs to learn how to run a well-organized meeting. Consider a few ground rules:

First, it must be short.

Second, it must end with action plans.

Third, it should be either informative/educational or action-oriented, although sometimes, both elements must be present.

Fourth, it must start and end on time, which shows respect for attendees. Early in my career as a CMO, another participant and I would join a meeting on time, but five others would not, so I would say, "Listen, let's hang on for three more minutes and give the others time to join."

I continued that practice until a physician challenged me, saying, "But *I* joined on time. Where are my three minutes? You're disrespecting my three minutes."

I never forgot that incident. Ever since, I have started my meetings on time, whether everyone has joined or not. I respect the folks who join on time, who therefore also show respect for me. And I've learned that the lesson catches on! Today, meeting participants join on time because they know we won't wait for them.

Fifth and finally, *never* have a meeting for the sake of a meeting, with no next steps. That disrespects everyone in the room.

Three Strategies for Good Time Management

Time management is crucial for a CMO because unexpected incidents constantly happen (e.g., you get a devastating call; somebody steps into your office with a serious problem; an emergency occurs in radiology). How can you run your schedule in a way that allows you to absorb these incidents without constantly chasing crises? I recommend three simple practices.

1. Prioritize your time through calendar management.

What must I do to keep myself sane and accomplish whatever needs to be done today? I constantly prioritize or delegate.

Suppose multiple meetings are scheduled to take place at the same time. Since I can't attend all three, I can choose to attend meeting A this month, while meeting B will have to wait until next month. And maybe I don't need to attend the third meeting at all.

I'm always working with my executive assistant, every week, to manage my calendar. "This one is a must meeting," I may say, "but this other one is a meeting that can wait. Please let the organizer of this one know that I may not be able to attend." Others can then chime in if I really need to attend. The weekly meeting with my assistant normally takes thirty minutes and saves *a lot* more time than that.

2. Don't take work home.

I don't take my work home unless I have no choice. Maintaining a clear boundary between my professional and personal life is essential for my executive well-being, as C-suite burnout is a genuine concern.

To the best of my ability, I try not to bring home to work either. To help with that, I use my office decorations as a visual reminder. I do not display pictures from home in my office. When questioned, I explain that I don't display my boss's picture at home, so why should I display home pictures at work? That's just me.

Of course, CMOs frequently get calls from work at odd hours; that is part of the job. Don't hesitate to share your contact information with your colleagues. I have found that the privilege is rarely, if ever, abused.

Nevertheless, practice drawing the line at *some* point in the day. Leave for tomorrow what can wait until the next day. At the end of any given day, I might have one hundred emails to which I need to respond. I quickly screen them, and if they can wait until the next day, they do so.

A Little Luck and a Lot of Hard Work

In the end, luck has little to do with becoming an effective CMO. For sure, luck has a hand in opening that window of opportunity to get your foot in the door! But once you're in, it is all hard work and building on your experiences.

Work hard on expanding your horizon beyond clinical medicine, and *never* shy away from investing in yourself. It is worth it, with or without the CMO role.

9

OTHER KEY CONSIDERATIONS

The topics in this chapter provide important additional information for all CMOs, new or established, to have in their armamentarium. It provides insights into effective high reliability principles, timing for career transitions, foundational real-life business knowledge, and unique challenges faced by female leaders.

High Reliability Organizations: CMO Leadership Is Key

Health care institutions across the country are in various stages of their journey toward becoming high reliability organizations. What does it mean to be a high reliability organization (HRO), and how can we translate this message to our medical staff and beyond? It may help to start with some history.

HRO theory is derived from normal accident theory, which led a group of researchers at the University of California, Berkeley, to study how organizations working with complex and hazardous systems operated error-free. The members of the group—Todd LaPorte, Gene Rochlin, and Karlene Roberts—researched three groups: United States nuclear aircraft carriers (in partnership with Rear Admiral (Ret.) Tom Mercer on the USS *Carl Vinson*); the Federal Aviation Administration's air traffic control system (and commercial aviation more generally); and nuclear power operations (Pacific Gas and Electric's Diablo Canyon reactor).

Although the original research and early application of HRO theory occurred in high-risk industries, the associated research covers a wide variety of applications and settings. Health care has been the largest practitioner area for the past several years.

Definition and Characteristics

A high reliability organization is an entity that operates in complex, high-risk environments while consistently maintaining safety and avoiding catastrophic failures. HROs are characterized by several key traits, including:

1. *A preoccupation with failure*: HROs are constantly on the alert for the potential of failure. They treat near misses as opportunities for learning and improvement.
2. *A reluctance to simplify*: HROs resist oversimplified explanations for problems, opting instead to dig deeper to understand the full context behind safety events.
3. *A sensitivity to operations*: HROs maintain a high level of awareness regarding their operations, ensuring that all employees are engaged in monitoring processes and systems.
4. A *commitment to resilience*: HROs are prepared to respond to unexpected challenges and recover quickly from errors or failures.
5. *A deference to expertise*: An HRO's decision-making is often based on expertise rather than hierarchy, allowing those with the most relevant knowledge to guide actions.

A 2024 book titled *High Reliability Healthcare*, by Dr. Jeffrey Kuhlman and Captain Robert Roncska, describes HRO principles and pillars in detail (I'll distinguish the two in a moment). The book asks a fundamental question: Why has the US Navy not suffered a single nuclear reactor disaster in more than seventy years of continuous operation, while health care continues to suffer from essentially the same percentage of adverse events that it did twenty-five years ago?

"High reliability health" became a rallying cry throughout the health care industry after the 1999 publication of a damning report from the Institute of Medicine called "To Err Is Human: Building a Safe Health System." It named medical errors as a leading cause of death in the United States and claimed most of them were preventable.

Two years later, a book by a pair of academics titled *Managing the Unexpected* laid out five principles of high reliability based on their study of high-profile accidents, primarily in the airline and oil industries. The health care industry rushed to adopt these principles . . . yet more than two decades later, the sad statistics regarding medical errors and patient harm simply have not improved. In fact, medical errors continue to rank among the top five causes of patient harm.

The numbers are staggering. More than seven *million* American patients are negatively impacted *each year* in some way by medical errors. Ten percent of patients in every American hospital will be part of some medication error. Every year, seven thousand to nine thousand Americans die from medical errors. These shocking statistics from *this* century underline the importance of high reliability operations. Patient safety is everyone's responsibility, and especially that of a CMO.

The safety of our patients depends on a combination of reliable systems and each of us individually committing ourselves to "doing the right thing" (both clinically and nonclinically). But what is that "right thing"? If the five high reliability principles of *Managing the Unexpected* haven't helped us to become the HROs we really want to be, then what will?

High Reliability Healthcare is a compelling and insightful resource that I recommend to professionals leading organizations in the pursuit of HRO status. The book differentiates between HRO principles and pillars. Principles focus on organizational culture, while pillars are viewed as personal accountabilities. In essence, HRO principles address upper management, while HRO pillars speak to the rank and file tasked with delivering health care services in person. This is where the divide exists between the cultures of the nuclear navy and contemporary health care.

The HRO pillars of the nuclear navy are embedded in the day-to-day activities of American seamen (a large percentage of whom are just eighteen to twenty years old), while the HRO pillars have only just begun to be introduced to clinicians, technicians, and other frontline workers in health care. *High Reliability Healthcare* describes the HRO pillars as follows:

1. *Higher understanding*

   We must have both a deep knowledge base, particularly related to our specific duties, as well as a broader understanding of our overall purpose. Suppose that nurse A, when asked about starting an IV line, says she's doing it because of a doctor's order. Nurse B, by contrast, explains she's starting it to treat septic shock and prevent harm to the patient. Can you guess who has a higher understanding of their role and is less likely to commit a medical error leading to harm?

2. *Integrity*

   This means we consistently choose to do what's right, regardless of the situation. Shared hand hygiene, for example, is critical in preventing hospital-acquired infections. We demonstrate integrity when everyone who enters a patient's room adheres to the hand hygiene protocol without exception.

3. *Formality*

   We comply with formal rules, use proper protocols, and refuse to bypass procedures. Time-outs and checklists exist for a reason. Can you imagine if surgeons failed to follow these protocols and policies in the operating room? Can you picture the potential patient harm as a result?

4. *Questioning attitude*

   This pillar calls us to be critical thinkers and seek better ways to accomplish tasks. Especially as CMOs, we must always encourage team members to think critically. Kuhlman and Roncska's book refers to the story of RaDonda Vaught, a former nurse found guilty in May 2022 of criminally negligent homicide and gross neglect of an impaired adult. Back in December 2017, she had injected a patient with the wrong medication, doing so by bypassing several safeguards and system warnings. The patient died the next day. Vaught was sentenced to three years of supervised probation with judicial diversion after facing up to eight years of imprisonment. She was also fired and lost her nursing license. I wonder, could questioning her manual override of a working system have prevented patient harm and kept her out of trouble?

5. *Backup*

   We look out for others by checking on our team members and providing assistance whenever needed. No one succeeds on an island. Effective health care involves collaboration. Team members must be provided with appropriate support in both positive and challenging circumstances.

Following organizational principles and individual pillars are both important in equipping a health care organization to become an HRO. Let me give one example of how HRO principles and pillars have worked together to keep our patients and associates safe.

A surgical team once called me to report that an operating surgeon was behaving oddly. I immediately sent another physician to oversee the surgery—remember, we do not compromise patient safety. We pulled the operating surgeon out to discuss the situation. The physician admitted to being under the influence of alcohol and was immediately placed on a leave of absence. Supported by colleagues at work and family members at home, the physician participated in a one-year intervention program, all of which was accomplished with complete confidentiality. Quarterly reports were carefully reviewed. One year later, the physician returned to work and produced excellent patient outcomes. This physician worked for two more years and then retired with dignity and grace. In this way, we assisted a colleague in a professional context while maintaining patient safety.

First, consider the HRO principles that worked well in this instance. In brief, the OR team was reluctant to simplify and refused to look for easy solutions. Instead, it deferred to expertise and so escalated to the CMO. Second, note the HRO pillars in action. The members of the OR team clearly understood their roles and recognized protocol breaches. The CMO responded promptly to support all involved. The physician showed integrity by enrolling in a program. Due to these quick interventions, patient care was not impacted and the team grew more resilient.

In situations like this, CMOs need to act quickly and with confidence. They must know the medical staff bylaws, be able to get a team together, understand the legal implications, and approach the situation with integrity.

The central question for us is this: How can HRO culture be ingrained throughout an organization so that every team member applies it consistently every day? At least five key strategies help to embed a culture of high reliability.

1. *Leadership development*: This includes the CEO! He/she also needs to be trained on the HRO principles and pillars.
2. *Culture of safety*: Don't play the blame game, but rather, provide psychological safety for staff to report events.
3. *Data systems*: Develop and use metrics that can be accurately measured and trended.
4. *Training and learning*: Constantly educate all staff members.

5. *Implement interventions*: Follow the PDSA quality improvement methodologies.

All physicians and team members need to be trained in HRO principles and pillars. These need to become ingrained in the fabric of the organization. Every team member must practice them in every action they take on the campus—without compromise.

The Timing of the Career Transition

What is the right time (if any) for a physician to explore leadership roles? Nearly all physicians, at one point in their career, will come to a fork in the road where they will question themselves. *Should I continue on this clinical path? Are there alternative places where I can perhaps learn and contribute even more?* Curiosity about significant administrative responsibilities will likely come calling at some point.

Some physicians, of course, have no desire to go down the administrative pathway, and that's okay too. Not all roles and responsibilities fit everyone. Many articles report that most physicians today have little interest in administrative leadership roles. They simply want to do shift work and then go home, and if that's their perspective and outlook, I say God bless 'em. We need these physicians right where they are. They serve a critical and necessary function, doing what they want to do and serving where they want to serve.

Still, I know there are many physicians, perhaps in their early-to-mid-fifties, who have begun to think, *I have ten more years left. Should I continue doing clinical, or should I do something different?* That's where I found myself in my early fifties, believing I needed to pursue an administrative track.

There are two basic tracks one can follow. In track one, you opt for dual responsibility. Clinical and administrative duties each get half of your time, which is perfectly fine for a medical directorship role. It is not possible, however, for a full-time chief medical officer position. To become a CMO, you must opt for track two. Why? The complexity and demands of the CMO role give physicians no time to continue any regular clinical duties. The myth that CMOs are better respected if they continue to do clinical is just that—a myth. Can you imagine the competency and skill set of any physician who does only one shift a month? The chances of patient harm go up steeply, compared to someone who does clinical for a living. The loss of clinical intuition (because not all of one's time is spent in clinical) undermines confidence and can negatively affect patient care, the very area the CMO position was created to improve.

I remember one CMO who would do one shift every other month in the ER. Team members soon shared their concerns about this arrangement with leadership. They found her to be ordering a lot more tests, taking a lot more time to assess, and having difficulty placing orders in the EMR. She was a capable physician, but without regular practice, any physician's skills can diminish, which compromises patient safety.

The time will come in your professional career when you must decide which path to follow. It will be a leap of faith. It is not easy, and it is a major decision for your professional career. Until then, you will have spent your entire career in clinical medicine, which becomes your identity. It is scary to let go of it! It truly takes a leap of faith, both in your own capabilities and in your belief that you can become an effective administrative leader. Worrying about whether you'd dislike the job or that you might fail in it often makes you hesitant to fully commit. I urge you to think differently. A hesitancy to fully commit to a role (especially one as important as CMO) can lead to making compromises or experiencing fatigue.

In my own time spent as a medical director and working as a clinical leader, I remember many instances when I found myself either shortchanging my administrative duties or not having meaningful conversations with my patients, who deserved my full attention. Once I made the choice to seek a CMO role, I enrolled in an MBA program while continuing to do full-time clinical. I completed my MBA in four and a half years, with the extra half-year to focus on maintaining my board certification. So, I skipped a semester, got board certified, and then continued my MBA. When I graduated, I had become a marketable candidate who could start applying for CMO roles.

Again, the timing of this move is extremely important. Few CMOs begin pursuing the role before completing fifteen years in their clinical careers. Most physicians graduate from their residency somewhere around their thirtieth birthday. While I've seen a thirty-nine-year-old CEO, I've never met a CMO that young.

For young physicians seeking to determine when in their careers they should begin considering a CMO role, my advice would be to start thinking about it early. Understand that this is not something taught in med school or residency. The conversations there always center on clinical or research topics; administrative skills are rarely mentioned. But if you think you may have what it takes, along with a real interest in it, then I believe it's important to start investigating early. Find your mentors and begin to identify your path early in your career. Approach it as any medical exam preparation that you undertake—research, prepare, and pass. Give yourself time to explore leadership roles and try them in small ways. Lead a project and get a taste of leading a team through relationships and building consensus. Only then will you be able to commit to this intense leadership role.

When I started exploring administrative leadership roles, my preparation included educating myself; I did not want to give up bedside clinical duties (which I loved) for something unknown. I began working with a mentor and participated in hospital committees and meetings. I had several CMO mentors, each with a distinct approach. I tried to take golden nuggets from each of them so that I could create my own style.

After years of working on committees and earning my MBA, I seized every chance to broaden my knowledge and better understand the field I intended to enter. As I've said, it's a similar approach to taking your board certification exams; you read, you learn, you prepare, and you attend preparation courses, all with the intention of passing. This exact mindset helped me prepare for the vast, unknown administrative enigma. I felt prepared, I had basic knowledge, and I had acquired the right skill set to succeed. I was ready.

Still, it took me a while. But when I finally made the decision to pursue an administrative career path, I went all in. Oh, yes, it felt daunting! I still miss patient interaction, but the clinical itch I continue to feel today is now addressed by serving in free health clinics, both locally and globally (that is another story for another day).

Foundational Knowledge

CMOs cannot impact the key performance indicators of a hospital without thoroughly understanding them. They therefore need to study and acquire knowledge in clinical documentation and care, revenue cycle, and utilization management. They also need to be proficient in and aware of various regulatory requirements, and they must become familiar with all laws that impact physician contracts. In addition, CMOs are the only ones who can connect the dots and explain the "why" to their own physician peers regarding the significance of documenting appropriately or the impact of transitioning patients at the right time. Only the CMO can clearly deliver these difficult messages.

In other words, a new CMO must have certain foundational knowledge to succeed in the role. CMOs don't need to be experts in all areas, but they must be significantly exposed to all the key elements of health care before taking on the role, including its business aspects.

Unfortunately, a few crucial elements of health care are never taught in med school or even in residency, *especially* the components related to business. These missing elements are nevertheless crucial for physicians to understand if they are to succeed in real-world practice and leadership roles.

For example, length of stay (LOS) is rarely talked about in residency. Medicare's DME and IME payments help residency programs nationwide to offset training costs. In practice, this metric can harm both patient and hospital finances if not managed appropriately. Why? Hospitals are paid by Medicare and many commercial payers using diagnosis-related groups (DRGs). Each DRG has a specific amount attached to it for a certain length of stay. Anything over that time will impact the hospital's bottom line. An increase in LOS of just half a day could amount to half a million dollars for the hospital. Longer LOS also exposes the patient to complications of being hospitalized, including infections, sarcopenia, or delirium, to name a few.

Managing LOS is a team sport that requires a skilled care management department collaborating closely with utilization management. Some hospitals hire physician advisors who counsel physicians in the trenches on care coordination and appropriate documentation. All these departments report to the chief medical officer.

At the end of the day, if the documentation does not support the medical necessity, insurance companies will deny payment to the hospital. Their decision will be reviewed by the revenue department, where the CMO is integral to helping craft process improvements and so decrease denials.

Hospital expenses grew by 5.1 percent in 2024, according to a recent brief from the American Hospital Association, outpacing the 2.9 percent inflation rate.[148] The brief also noted that labor costs are the biggest driver, with advertised nursing salaries rising 26.6 percent faster than inflation from 2020 to 2024. Hospitals want to recoup such costs through operational efficiencies—and the one metric that encapsulates it all is LOS.

Health systems are also increasingly suing insurance companies over disputes related to payment issues, contract negotiations, and claim denials. When hospitals and insurance companies have disagreements, patients often find themselves caught in the middle. They may pay more, experience care delays, or need to change providers.

In New York City, negotiations between UnitedHealthcare and Memorial Sloan Kettering Cancer Center missed a June 30, 2025, deadline, which briefly left some patients in limbo until a deal was reached the next day.[149] In North Carolina, Duke Health announced it could leave the Aetna network unless the insurance company agreed to pay more favorable rates to the health system, which could have placed many patients out of network for their physicians and made them liable for payment. Fortunately for all involved, the two reached a new agreement in late 2025.[150] For three months, Anthem patients in Missouri lost access to in-network care at the region's largest (and sometimes sole) medical provider due to a dispute between insurers and the health system. Indeed, 18 percent of nonfederal hospitals experienced at least one documented case of public brinkmanship with an insurance company from June 2021 to May 2025, according to preliminary findings by Jason Buxbaum, a health policy researcher at the Brown University School of Public Health. Over the same period, 8 percent of hospitals ultimately went out-of-network with an insurer, at least for a time.[151]

A federal law dubbed the No Surprises Act, which took effect in 2022, offers protections for some patients whose provider drops out of network due to a contract dispute.[152] Individuals getting treatment for serious conditions can keep their in-network rates for up to ninety days with their current providers, delaying the need to find a new one or face higher rates.

Keep in mind that this is just *one* example of the myriad business issues that deeply affect the delivery of safe, effective health care. In a book titled *The Hidden Power of Relentless Stewardship*, Don Jernigan, the late CEO of Adventist Health System (now AdventHealth), wrote some powerful words that resonate deeply with me:

> The fact is that much of the looseness, sloppiness, and poor performance that plagues many not-for-profits develops because people within these organizations don't grasp the legitimate relationship between mission and money. That is, they don't understand the concept of stewardship. But you do yourself and your organization no moral good by divorcing mission and money. Both secular and faith-based

> not-for-profits need to be as strong and disciplined about this issue as any for-profit group in the world.[153]

The CMO should stay informed about these real-life examples. Reading journals, attending conferences, and giving public presentations all add to our foundational knowledge cache.

A Word to Female Physician Leaders

As I worked on this project, I quickly recognized how infrequently female CMOs have authored works in this field. This, of course, made me more determined than ever to get this book published.

This chapter is not an attempt to address gender bias or leadership in general—these are complex social issues that require broader discussion. But I did want to speak to female physician leaders and dedicate a segment of my book to this crucial discussion.

The fact is that a different subset of core competencies applies to female leaders, irrespective of their profession. If you are a woman, I have no doubt that you can relate to this statement! But what must female physician leaders do that differs from their male counterparts?

Let me begin my answer by saying that I do not want to spin this negatively and talk only about the obstacles. I would much rather discuss what women need to do and how they can shine in this complex world of medical leadership. Gender bias in leadership continues to exist even in this decade. The big irony is that the impact it has on the individual and on the organization often continues to go unrecognized.

Studies have shown that such a potent image of male versus female leadership has been created over centuries that by now it has been imprinted on our subconscious. When either gender deviates from this common cognitive imprint, a bias is created in the psyche of most observers. I remember rounding with my residents. Many times, patients would address my male resident as the attending. That is the societal mindset. A male leader who is quiet and agreeable may be seen as lacking authority, while a female leader who is assertive may be considered abrasive. Both conclusions are incorrect, and that is how cognitive bias works. Our job is to recognize it within ourselves and be intentional about removing it from our decision-making processes.

Studies have shown that women in general fail to recognize subtle discrimination. This is an important fact that I would like medicine's future female leaders to focus on and address. Don't normalize words like "honey" or "sweetheart," regardless of who uses them in the workplace. Do not hesitate to call it out and address it as inappropriate. Your actions will help build your colleagues' insight and begin to resolve the issue much faster.

In 2020, women held only 29 percent of senior management positions globally. It's even more difficult for a woman to climb that wall in organizations that have predominantly hierarchical structures. A 2021 article in *JAMA* states:

> Although women currently represent a slight majority of the US population and a large majority of the US health care workforce,[154] they are generally underrepresented on leadership teams, which likely diminishes their role in policy decisions that affect population and women's health. . . . Women [hold] only approximately 15% of the CEO positions in health care organizations.[155]

A white paper published online by San Francisco–based health care startup supporter Rock Health reports that women make up 18 percent of US hospital CEOs and 4 percent of health care company CEOs. Iya Khalil, the co-founder and executive vice president of GNS Healthcare, declared, "I believe the lack of women executive leaders (in terms of numbers compared to men) is due to not having enough role models and women not knowing what they can achieve in this space." I agree with her assessment, and I hope this book provides insight for any courageous female physician leaders who choose a future career as a chief medical officer.

In the United States, 35.5 percent of CMOs are women, which translates to approximately 12,519 female CMOs currently employed in the health care sector. That figure is up from 31.48 percent in 2010. This is progress! But we still have a long way to go.

It may help here to recognize that female physicians have significantly shaped the field of medicine. We stand on the shoulders of a great number of female physicians from the past who made groundbreaking contributions to the world of medicine. Let me recall just a few.[156]

Elizabeth Blackwell was the first woman in the United States to earn an MD degree (in 1849!). She went on to become the founder of the New York Infirmary for Women and Children and establish a medical college for women.

Rebecca Lee Crumpler became the first African American woman to earn an MD degree (in 1864!). In her younger years, she often accompanied her aunt on trips to care for sick neighbors. These experiences inspired her to go into medicine. She described these trips and their influence on her in a book she published in 1883. She became a pioneer in medicine and a key figure in the fight for women's rights in the medical field.

Mary Edwards Walker was a surgeon during the Civil War, a women's rights advocate, an abolitionist, a spy, and the only woman in US history to receive the Medal of Honor (which the government took away in 1916. President Jimmy Carter legally restored it in 1977). In 1871, she published her own book, *Hit: Essays on Women's Rights*, a partly autobiographical work.

Patricia Bath was a pioneer in ophthalmology and the first Black woman to receive a medical patent, which she earned for her invention of the laserphaco probe, a device created to improve cataract surgery.

Antonia Novello was the first Hispanic woman to serve as the US surgeon general, serving from 1990 to 1993. In her role as surgeon general, she prioritized pediatric AIDS awareness, neonatal care, and anti-smoking campaigns geared toward youth.

Katalin Karikó, a Hungarian-American biochemist, laid the scientific groundwork for mRNA vaccines. In 2023, she received the Nobel Prize in Physiology or Medicine for her pioneering work.

These are just a few of the outstanding women in health care who have brought us to where we are today. The historical narrative of women in medicine resonates with perseverance, brilliance, and profound yet often unappreciated impact. From the revolutionary efforts of historical women in medicine, such as Crumpler and Walker, to modern pioneers, such as Novello and Karikó, women in science and medicine have continuously shaped health care for the better. I hope my own book inspires young female physicians to pursue leadership and build their own identity.

Avoid limiting yourself to predefined categories! Your style will differ from that of others, which is great, because *you* are different. Female leaders must be sharp, well presented, rational, and committed to their leadership path. Learn to view adversities as challenges. Face the sunshine so the shadows will fall behind you. And don't give up! The future of female physician leaders is very bright, indeed.

A Challenge Worth Accepting

The critical role of the chief medical officer has evolved tremendously in the last ten years. And it continues to change! Yes, it can be a challenge, but for those who want to shape health care for the better, it's a challenge well worth accepting.

Physician leadership is essential in this ever-evolving health care world that is becoming more complex as time goes on. New technologies on the horizon pose an ethical dilemma for our clinicians. Questions around artificial intelligence are growing rapidly, even as I write this chapter. It is increasingly important for physicians to assume leadership roles and thus actively contribute to the advancement of modern medicine. If we opt out of decision-making, we forfeit the right to complain.

Chief medical officers are uniquely positioned to lead our physicians and executive suites across the world, thus contributing toward high-quality, safe care for our patients. Do not shy away from this role. Make it your purpose and calling.

Remind yourself that no CMO works in a vacuum; health care is a team sport. See this as a challenge and an opportunity. Learn to work in a matrix system and partner with the CNO for bedside clinical care, the COO for equipment needs, and the CFO for contracts. And of course, work with the CEO to help guide the vision of your organization.

The chief medical officer position is one of the most challenging executive roles because it relies almost solely on influence. Perhaps for that very reason, it is a challenge worth accepting. It's also one of the most rewarding jobs imaginable, as it profoundly impacts patients' lives. It is worth it! And you can make it your own.

10

SOME COLLEGIAL COUNSEL

In preparing to write this book, I interviewed many medical professionals to get their perspectives on working with chief medical officers. In their view, what makes a good CMO? How can they be most effective? What traits or characteristics are essential?

Most of their comments are spread throughout the book, but I believe it might be helpful for readers to hear some of their comments that didn't necessarily "fit" in a specific chapter. In this appendix, therefore, I present some additional insight and perspective from leaders that you may find instructive, encouraging, and helpful.

As in the rest of the book, I name the two CEOs quoted and preserve the anonymity of the other contributors. All comments have been lightly edited for clarity.

Ken Lukhard, Former Hospital CEO, Now Retired

When I arrived at one hospital, it was a large, bloated, poorly run organization. It was full, partly because the length of stay was very high and because doctors were all doing their own thing. The hospital was not making a lot of money based on its size and its patient base, so we totally redefined what that organization was going to become. We said, "We want to become one of the best major teaching hospitals in the country." We wanted to compare ourselves to hospitals that people didn't want to compete with. The first step was to become a major teaching hospital.

We *were* a teaching hospital at the time, but our data was not compared to the major teaching hospitals because it was in a different category. The chief medical officer at that time did a really good job leading the charge to get us into that category of major teaching hospitals. First, we had to expand our scope. All the infrastructure that had to be built, like the recruitment of doctors and the building of programs. That's a task that I couldn't *begin* to do. *He* had to do it, and he did it really, really well.

Once we got into that bucket, there was the challenge of competing effectively, in a clinical sense, with those other organizations. That was the goal: to be as clinically sound or better than the academic medical centers that were all major teaching hospitals. So, we got our designation as a major teaching hospital. And then we were being compared to the big centers.

We quickly found out that our health outcomes were not nearly what they should have been. An article published early in my tenure in an area newspaper said we were at the top of the list of the worst-performing hospitals, clinically. That was a wake-up call. I hadn't been there very long when that hit the newspaper.

We found an ED physician who was really bright and had a lot of innate skills. I sat down with him a few times and asked him about his interest in becoming a leader in the organization. "Yeah, I would be interested," he said. He had gone to business school and had earned a business degree as well.

We had one bundle of health outcomes that was not doing well compared to the other places in the city. We paired that ED physician with a nurse leader, our director of quality, and the two formed a dyad. They went after that bundle. They came in and, at first, they reported every two weeks, then once a month. In less than one year, we went from being at the eighth percentile to the ninety-third percentile. It was all because this physician led that charge. Yes, he had a dyad partner, and they made a great team.

So, if he did that with one bundle, I said to him, "Would you be interested in leaving the emergency room and becoming a full-time leader?"

"Absolutely," he said. That's how his career went. He ended up becoming our vice president of clinical innovation. I bragged about him so much that they hired him at the corporate office, and then he got hired away. Now he's the CEO of a big health system.

The point is that you must make those kinds of improvements from a quality standpoint—improvements in clinical services, developing and implementing quality clinical metrics, things like that. That all falls within the purview of a CMO. That's what this guy did, and he did it superbly.

One day, I was sitting with Fawn Lopez, the long-time former editor in chief of *Modern Healthcare*. She's a very well-known lady. We were at a big event with the annual top one hundred hospitals. They break those one hundred into the top fifteen major teaching hospitals, and then the top fifteen large community hospitals, and so on down to the best little hospitals. I was there representing our hospital to receive an award for being one of the top major teaching hospitals. By that time, we were a few years down the road, having gone from the eighth percentile of the country to being in the top fifteen hospitals in the country. We were being compared to places like Johns Hopkins and Stanford—the premier group. By then, we were in their company.

"Ken," Fawn said to me, "you've done an amazing job. You haven't been there all that long, and all of a sudden, coming out of nowhere, you've done all this. How have you done it?"

"Well, Fawn," I replied, "without the leadership of a physician executive, we wouldn't be here today. There's no way."

Once the organization was thriving, we brought in a new chief medical officer, Dr. Rick Scott. We saw that one of our areas of vulnerability was related to our expansion of the campus. We built a bed tower and an ambulatory building. The expansion cost a billion dollars. It was amazing. But even as we expanded our ICU capability, our ICUs were full all the time. We had around 150 different kinds of ICU beds: cardiac beds, neuro beds, and so forth. Some of the units, like the cardiac ICU units, were run by the surgical group. They provided their own intensivists. But the generic ICUs did not have twenty-four-hour coverage on the floor.

Rick said to me, "You know, to be elite, we've got to get twenty-four-hour intensivists on those ICU floors." Doctors didn't like it at first. They'd say, "You're cutting into our hours."

"You know," we said, "this is about patient care, outcomes, patient safety, and quality improvement." Over some months, we sold them on that idea. Rick then developed a model that became the advocate standard. We hired a bunch of great doctors—really well-trained, young, bright, rock stars—to run the ICUs as full-time intensivists. The quality of care and outcomes improved dramatically. It was just awesome.

The CEO of a Legacy Hospital in Illinois

Most physicians and clinicians, including me, have a bias toward action. I once worked with a CMO who carried around a pocket pad and a pen. If this CMO wrote it down in her little book, it would happen. The loop was closed, the issue was solved, and everything was tied in a bow. It was done. She was great.

I worked with another CMO who believed that a conversation could fix anything. He thought we had to expand the pool of knowledge and meaning, and we'd do that by getting around the table to define and create how we might accomplish something together. "So, how might we reduce length of stay by X number of days in the next month?" "How might we improve our first case on-time starts in the OR?" He got the teams together and expanded on that pool of knowledge and meaning, and he got everybody focused on where we could head.

But the best of the best have a bias toward action. They drive performance and move the team along while forming relationships along the way.

When you're a chief medical officer, you are now a strategy builder, a planner, an executor, and a responsible member of the executive cabinet. Some CMOs will say, "Well, I'm just medical staff. This is my room. If it involves a physician, I'm there." No. The best CMOs understand where they fit in the whole spectrum, the whole picture, the whole strategy and performance and operations of the hospital, from the cafe to the OR to parking and back again. They understand how they're visible in the community, their environment, and all aspects of the executive team.

When I am looking to hire a CMO, I'm always looking at things such as what their influences are, how they handle problems, how they innovate and strategize with a team, and whether they're liked and respected by their peers. If I don't know someone, I want to get to know them as a person. I want to ensure that they're aligned with our mission and culture, that they have a collaborative spirit, and that they have proof of strategic and financial acumen and good communication skills and interactions. You can tell a lot in the interview process, making sure that the candidate is flexible, isn't resistant to change.

I like to ask fun interview questions, and they're *so* telling. My first question is, "If you're stranded on a deserted island, what three things would you bring with you and why?" The answer to that question speaks volumes about the individual. If someone replies, "I'd bring a book, a glass of iced tea, and my La-Z-Boy," that tells me they're probably not going to have a bias toward action. They're not thinking about strategy and longevity; they're just waiting to see what happens as they sip their tea. I've ruled out candidates using this question.

A thoughtful person may say, "Let me think about it." They don't think too long before saying, "I would have to bring a source to create fire." And then they go through various things—usually, it's a water source, a fire source, and something for protection. You get all kinds of answers with this question.

A lot of people will say, "Can I ask a question about the island?" I love that because it shows they're inquisitive. They're not just jumping to the answers.

Some people realize later they have answered badly, then come back and email me their new answers. I have had that happen. I didn't hire that person.

A second question I sometimes ask is this: "If I were to look into your closet, what would I see?" Oftentimes, you'll learn about people's hobbies. They'll say, "I have a ton of ski equipment there," and then you can say, "Oh okay. Do you ski?" And you can get into the skiing conversation. You know they're risk-takers, those types of things.

Highly organized people often say, "My winter clothes are here, and my spring clothes are over there," while others admit, "My closet is a mess." And then I think, *No, not a doer*. They have no attention to detail. They're lackadaisical.

I use these two questions continually, and they have never failed me. They assist my decision when I'm unsure if I've truly understood someone. They're very helpful.

Allen Verrill, the CEO of a Large Health Care Organization in the Midwest (He Likes to Call Himself "The Recovering CMO"!)

I think CMOs need to strive to be the best in class.

I'm a physician by training and experience. I still believe that everything about me is oriented toward the clinician's world. People ask me, "Do you enjoy being a CEO?" And I say, "Yes, it's been a growth orientation for me that has been very positive in my life." But it was never my aspiration to be an administrator.

I have over twenty years of clinical medicine experience as my background. I'm an internist, and I cut my teeth on hospital medicine back in the day when hospital medicine was just forming. I graduated from medical school more than thirty years ago.

My real pathway into leadership started when I took a US Air Force scholarship for medical school. I spent eleven years on active duty as part of my military application after medical school, if you add the four years of medical school where I wore the uniform intermittently, like for the training I used to have in the summers, and then the seven years I wore it every day, three of which were my residency. The military combined all the aspects of what I needed to do to train for a career as a physician after medical school and then added the whole military experience onto it. I'm a strong introvert; I really had never led anything. But when you're an officer in the military, you wear the leadership experience. They used to say, "You're an officer first and foremost. You're a physician second." Now, I'm not sure those of us who were physicians fully believed that, but there was some truth to it.

During that time, I treated some VIPs, usually four-star generals or their families. That's a unique type of medicine. I discovered there's a real difference between being a commander and a leader.

In the midst of that, I learned more about myself and got comfortable with some leadership skills. Then I transitioned to a civilian practice, where there were problems that needed to be solved in the hospital group that employed me. I worked for a hospital system back in Maine, and the problems that I was asked to engage in affected my practice. I had developed some experience at those tables because the military forced me into those places, which made me willing to say yes when I was volunteered or asked to be a volunteer in those spaces. They didn't seem like that big of a deal to me; I was trying to help my practice improve. I didn't recognize at the time that the pathway was one you could do more formally. You could help train people to have some leadership experience and problem-solving experience, above and beyond the clinical experience. I think we're better at that today than we were in my early career. After a while, I became a hospitalist and helped build and run the hospitalist practice.

I became a CMO in 2015 in Colorado, where I was recruited after about twenty years of clinical practice, fifteen of which were in the civilian world in Maine. I did a little bit of clinical practice in Colorado for a couple of years, and then slowly, I gave up practice. I last saw patients around 2017. And then in 2020, COVID-19 hit. I helped run incident command. It was a very intense time.

About seven or eight months into running that incident command, my former boss contacted me to see if I had any interest in being a CEO and helping open a new hospital in 2021, a year from the time he was calling me. He told me he was specifically looking to hire a physician leader to help build and grow the medical staff at the new hospital. He thought a physician leader would be great. I hadn't really considered being a CEO, but it made me pause to say, "Okay, if I were to become a CEO at a new hospital, with a new medical staff and all new structures, I would be the one to help build it. I might be able to get my hands around what that means from a CEO standpoint. I would understand some of the dynamics from a business and operational standpoint that might be able to make me successful as a CEO, even though that's never guaranteed."

I talked to my coach and to a few other people and then threw my hat in. I took that job, which I did for the better part of four years. Then my boss invited me to come up to a five-hundred-bed hospital, well-established for over sixty years, to help lead there. Now I'm at a full-scale hospital—not a new hospital, but one that has a long legacy. I feel like I've built a résumé of CEO experience that's allowed me to be remotely capable of entering this space.

Maybe the best example of achieving clarity of communication through repeated communications happened during COVID-19. When we opened our incident command during COVID-19, we had honestly no idea what we were dealing with. It was one of the first times clinically I've ever experienced—and probably the only time clinically on a broad scale—where we had something that we knew was going to be serious. As we came closer and closer to having actual COVID-19 patients hit our facility, we had no idea about the risk to individual clinicians, meaning all of us sitting at the hospital, at some level. We had no real idea how to treat this. It was a learning lab, and we knew that to protect ourselves, we probably needed a bunch of equipment that we didn't have.

We were constantly making clinical decisions that were incomplete, based on insufficient information. They all affected our clinical operations. We set up an incident command center run by CMOs. CMOs were running our clinical operations, which took over most of our hospital operations. We iterated time and time again with what we knew and what we didn't know.

So, they were open to saying, "We're going to re-engage in this conversation at regular intervals and update you." It became the science of communication during that time.

We had huddles at the local and system level two, sometimes three, times a day. Because the flow of communication was so dynamic and so uncertain and so great and changed so often, we became professionals and experts at communicating the unknown. We got pretty darn good at that.

A system CMO led the charge at that time. She did a fantastic job. She set up and organized the whole system, making sure that it was connected. We ended up having all our hospitals report at the huddle daily. We had all our CMOs engaging with the various questions they were facing. I think it was the best in a very uncertain world.

That time provided a reminder to us all: Leadership is most important when it's the toughest. When the decisions are hardest and feel the worst, when you go home at night unsure of your choices because the situation is complex and affects people's lives, that's when leadership is the most important. A lot of physician leaders want to step back and either delegate that responsibility or step away from it altogether. But that's when I believe leadership is the absolute most important—when you need to be in the thick of it, to work through those times with patience and repetitive communication. It's also where, a lot of times, I see people wanting to pull the rip cord and bail out. I remind them that's the *exact* time when their leadership is most trying yet most important.

You think of the examples of the Lincolns or the Churchills of the world. They shone most when times were absolutely dire and it looked like nothing was ever going to work. You don't know how it's all going to work out when you're in the middle of it, but leaders *stay* in the middle of it.

A Chief Nursing Officer

Probably the most difficult time my CMO and I dealt with was COVID-19. I wanted to keep my staff safe, even with everybody pushing everything on nursing. For example, dietary aides didn't want to walk into rooms, so bedside nurses were donning and delivering meals. The CMO and I were so close during those months of uncharted territory. During the first three months, *nobody* knew what they were doing. Toward the end, when we were getting tired and working seven days a week with little or no rest, it was the CMO who held the physicians together, who could explain the ever-evolving pandemic scientifically to the staff. I believe it was our strong dyad partnership that was key during those critical times.

Resiliency had such a huge role to play during a time of great uncertainty. The CMO was constantly on the phone with doctors, talking to them and telling them, "This is all we know right now. This is what the CDC is telling us to do. We have to follow this. We have to go with that." It was surreal to see the choices that our clinicians had to make. It was a difficult time, and that's when leadership counts the most.

From a Director of Risk

I think CMOs should listen, be open to trying new things, and connect with frontline staff and nursing leaders. When the staff tries to speak to doctors about some issue, they often feel that their comments go into a black hole. It's helpful if the chief medical officer is rounding on the units, working with nursing leaders and staff, and reassuring them that their concerns related to the medical staff will be taken seriously. They see that and know their CMO wants to help them.

I'm a clinician by background. I know what it's like when certain doctors are on shift and working. They're not easy to talk to. If you have a concern that you try to bring to that provider and you get ignored, you want to feel empowered to go to your CMO for assistance. You want your CMO to be available, approachable, and open, not defensive.

A Regional Director of Quality and Patient Safety

I think one of the key attributes of a successful CMO is a deep understanding of regulatory requirements, including those from the Centers for Medicare and Medicaid Services and Leapfrog. Other key attributes include embracing patient safety and being open-minded as they work to balance cost with efficiency and safety. Embracing patient safety is a crucial attribute for any CMO, including being transparent and open about areas needing improvement. A CMO must also be able to participate in disclosure discussions with patients when things do not go as planned, in this way demonstrating both transparency and vulnerability. Good CMOs also know how to coach physicians on how to have difficult conversations with patients, an important factor in improving patient safety and being mindful of risk management.

A Young Physician Considering a Future in Leadership

My goal moving forward in leadership is mainly to go into the quality realm or any role that makes an impact. Whether that means becoming a CMO or a chief quality officer, I'm not sure. I'm still trying to figure that out. It depends on what the role offers and especially on what kind of impact I might have. My CMO and I have had this conversation. I've always looked up to her as my mentor. I've always told her, "I don't know if I want to be a CMO. I have other interests." But if I do get the opportunity to be a CMO in a place where I can impact greater changes, then yes, I would probably look into that.

I had a lot of mentors where I did my master's in health care quality. I keep in touch with some of them to this day as I try to figure out my path. If one day I were to become a mentor to someone on a similar path, I would say to them, "Start with the question of knowing your 'why.' Why do you want this direction? If you don't understand the 'why,' it's hard to go down that path. Is it just that you want an administrative position? Or is it because you want to make an impact? Are you thinking you want to do 50/50, clinical and administrative?" That all helps determine your path.

Once they decide that, I think I would slowly mentor them, step by step, just like what my CMO did with me: "Let's expose you to those little committees, little day-to-day activities, to see if you feel comfortable taking a little bit of ownership. We'll go from there." And of course, I'd also tell them to look into all these leadership courses and certifications so that they know some basics before getting that role.

* * *

Do you see a common thread in these conversations? I do. These are either seasoned leaders, very advanced in their leadership journey, or physicians aspiring to greater leadership positions. But they all have one common goal: They desire to positively impact patient care. They all arrived at their destinations having traveled varied paths, but the common "why" for all was to move their institutions to be the best in delivering good clinical care.

I can't thank them enough for taking the time to speak with me and for being willing to share their expertise in this book. I do hope I have done justice to their thoughts! If not, I also know they will read this with a smile, nodding in agreement . . . and definitely with grace.

Epilogue

YOU'RE UP TO THE TASK

A few years into my CMO role, one physician's actions caught me off guard. As a member of the board, she made a disparaging remark about me in my absence. When I asked her for feedback and the context surrounding her comment, she replied, "Oh, I heard it from someone else. I wasn't there in the meeting myself." It immediately struck me that she had remembered an offhand comment from another colleague, made it her own, and then repeated it at a high-level meeting.

I tell this story because such a scenario *will* happen to you at some point in your own leadership journey. I once read a quote by billionaire executive Warren Buffett that caught my eye: "You will continue to suffer if you have an emotional reaction to everything that is said to you. True power is sitting back and observing things with logic. True power is restraint. If words control you, that means everyone else can control you. Breathe and allow things to pass." It is sage advice, but it's oh-so-difficult to practice! The conversation I had with that physician kept me up one whole night, reflecting on how I could improve and reminding myself not to take her comment personally.

Leadership roles are lonely, so be prepared to be both disappointed and hurt by your colleagues. But guess what? You will do the same to them (and be criticized for it). This is inevitable, so prepare yourself mentally.

In my view, the best answer is to lead with grace. Give grace to yourself as a leader and extend grace toward others. This is the only way I know to spark both kindness and understanding. While you shouldn't expect it to be reciprocated all the time, you can certainly practice it yourself.

The road from stethoscope to boardroom is both arduous and long. It will challenge your resolve. You will find yourself questioning your decision to become a chief medical officer. My advice? Go find your battle buddy, build a small and mighty support group, and remember that this path is not merely a choice but a calling.

Remember, too, that C-suite burnout is real. Don't give up! It is our privilege and our duty to lead the quality and safety journey for our patients. Remember that physicians are uniquely qualified to lead in this way, for several reasons. We can readily become capable, effective, and knowledgeable leaders because of our inherent characteristics, our position, our effectiveness as change agents, and our innate understanding of the front lines of care. Every chief medical officer has lived on the front lines, understands what it takes to deliver care, and can translate this knowledge into the administrative corridor. We possess both clinical expertise and the capability to take the lead.

So, as you continue this journey, I urge you to adopt a team leader approach. Remain dedicated to patient safety, and increase your emotional intelligence—it will only enhance your effectiveness as a change agent.

Let me end this book by paraphrasing the Hippocratic oath that all of us as physicians swear to uphold. Though not adapted specifically for leadership roles, it can serve as the foundation for ethical leadership. My adaptation emphasizes the importance of patient welfare, respect for human life, and a commitment to continuous learning.

Let's continue to be the light for the only real task of every CMO: the delivery of high-quality health care and patient safety. That's our job.

And yes, you're up to the task.

THANK YOU NOTE

I am deeply grateful to the many colleagues who generously shared their time, perspectives, and insights. Their thoughtful contributions are woven throughout this book, enriching its content and enhancing its credibility. Their expertise brought depth to these pages and helped ground the work in the lived realities of physician leadership.

To past chief medical officers: Thank you for laying the foundation upon which today's physician leaders stand.

To current CMOs: Your courage to lead with integrity, navigate complexities, and prioritize what matters most is both inspiring and essential.

To those preparing to step into the role of CMO: I extend my sincere best wishes. Let patient safety and the well-being of those we serve remain your unwavering North Star.

I wish to acknowledge my collaborative author, Steve Halliday. His ability to distill and organize the insights of so many distinguished leaders was key in bringing this book to life.

To Dr. Kuhlman: Thank you for writing the foreword and for your guidance throughout this journey. Your steady encouragement, wisdom, and support have been instrumental every step of the way.

Finally, to my family: Thank you for your unwavering support and ongoing patience—always.

ABOUT THE AUTHOR

Dr. **Bela Nand, MD, MBA** is the vice president and chief medical officer for the Advent Health Mid-America Region, where she provides executive leadership for clinical quality, patient safety, and physician engagement across a multihospital system. In this role, she partners closely with physicians and administrative leaders to advance high reliability care, strengthen medical staff governance, and deliver measurable improvements in outcomes and patient experience.

Dr. Nand earned her medical degree and went on to complete postgraduate training in internal medicine. She further advanced her leadership expertise by completing a master of business administration, strengthening her capabilities in health care strategy, finance, and organizational leadership. She is board certified in internal medicine, hospice and palliative medicine and has completed Lean Six Sigma Green Belt training, reflecting her commitment to performance improvement and operational excellence.

With a career spanning clinical practice and executive leadership, Dr. Nand is recognized for driving system-wide transformation through data-informed decision-making and collaborative physician leadership models. She has led numerous initiatives focused on quality improvement, patient safety, and operational performance, aligning multidisciplinary teams around shared goals of accountability and continuous improvement.

A dedicated advocate for physician leadership development, Dr. Nand has been instrumental in designing and advancing programs that prepare physicians to lead effectively in evolving health care systems. Her work emphasizes the integration of clinical expertise with administrative acumen, particularly through dyad leadership frameworks.

Dr. Nand's leadership philosophy is grounded in professionalism, integrity, and lifelong learning. She remains committed to advancing the role of physicians as leaders in health care and mentoring the next generation of physician executives.

ENDNOTES

1 Nicholas Chadi, "Medical Leadership: Doctors at the Helm of Change," *McGill Journal of Medicine* (1): 52–57, January 12, 2009, bing.com/ck/a?!&&p=c0d-d335cf528c3e36ea65e38e04af245eb75b613d95977a-7adb34d0b7aa4adfbJmltdHM9MTc1OTEwNDAwMA&p-tn=3&ver=2&hsh=4&fclid=12e48fc7-97f9-6d21-13f2-9aaa-96436c9e&psq=Nicholas+Chadi%2c+Medical+Leadership%3a+-Doctors+at+the+Helm+of+Change%2c+Mcgill+J+Med&u=a-1aHR0cHM6Ly9tam0ubWNnaWxsLmNhL2FydGljbGUvZG9-3bmxvYWQvNzM0LzUzMy8yMzMz&ntb=1.

2 Mariah Taylor, "Split physician roles in action: A guide from AMCs," *Becker's Clinical Leadership*, July 25, 2025, https://www.beckershospitalreview.com/quality/hospital-physician-relationships/split-physician-roles-in-action-a-guide-from-amcs/.

3 Ibid.

4 Ibid.

5 Ibid.

6 David Nash, "Who's at the Helm? The Evolving Role of the Physician Executive," *MedPage Today*, January 3, 2023, https:/www.medpagetoday.com/opinion/focus-on-policy/102480.

7 Caren Fleit, "The Evolution of the CMO," *Harvard Business Review,* July–August 2017, https://hbr.org/2017/07/the-evolution-of-the-cmo.

8 "The Evolution of Physician Leadership: From Lone Healers to Integral Hospital Managers in Modern Healthcare," Simbo AI, accessed March 17, 2026, https://www.simbo.ai/blog/the-evolution-of-physician-leadership-from-lone-healers-to-integral-hospital-managers-in-modern-healthcare-659039.

9 American Hospital Association, *Advancing Health*, "The Evolving Role of the Physician Leader," January 9, 2024, https:/www.aha.org/advancing-health=podcast/2024-01-10-evolving-role-physician-leader.

10 Kathy Matzka, "Negligent Credentialing Lawsuits: Case Law Examples," *Symplr*, July 19, 2016, https://www.symplr.com/blog/negligent-credentialing-lawsuits-case-law-examples.

11 Ibid.

12 "Hospital Negligent Credentialing: Legal Challenges and Patient Safety," Brewster & De Angelis Advocates, June 4, 2024, https://www.brewsterlaw.com/hospital-negligent-credentialing-legal-challenges-and-patient-safety.

13 Fleit, op. cit.

14 Nash, op. cit.

15 American Hospital Association, op. cit.

16 Chadi, p. 52.

17 Chadi, p. 53.

18 Chadi, p. 53.

19 Chadi, p. 54.

20 Nash, op. cit.

21 Fleit, op. cit.

22 Martha Sonnenberg, "Changing Roles and Skill Sets for Chief Medical Officers," *American Association of Physician Leaders*, June 19, 2018, https://www.physicianleaders.org/articles/changing-roles-skill-sets-chief-medical-officers.

23 Sonnenberg, op. cit.

24 Sonnenberg, op. cit.

25 Ibid.

26 Sonnenberg, op. cit.

27 Sonnenberg, op. cit.

28 Nash, op. cit.

29 "Job outlook for chief medical officers in the United States," Zippia, accessed March 17, 2026, https://www.zippia.com/chief-medical-officer-jobs/trends.

30 Ibid.

31 Peter B. Angood, "Physician Leadership: More Valuable Than Ever—A White Paper from the American Association for Physician Leadership," September 2022, page 2, www.physicianleaders.org/articles/doi/10.55834.wp.9897031832.

32 Ibid., p. 17.

33 Christopher G. Myers, Daniel Polsky, and Sanjay Desai, "The Growing Role of Chief Medical Officers in Major Corporations," *JAMA Health Forum*, July 22, 2022, https://jamanetwork.com/journals/jama-health-forum/fullarticle/2794537.

34 Nick Henderson, "Preparing the Next Generation of Chief Medical Officers in an Evolving Landscape," Russell Reynolds Associates, October 9, 2023, https://www.russellreynolds.com/en/insights/reports-surveys/preparing-the-next-generation-of-chief-medical-officers-in-an-evolving-landscape.

35 Ibid.

36 AHRQ 2011.

37 Ibid.

38 Interview with director of risk, June 9, 2025. The name of the interviewee is withheld by mutual agreement.

39 Francesca Mathewes, "The evolution of the chief medical officer," *Becker's Physician Leadership*, June 24, 2025, https://www.beckersphysicianleadership.com/chief-medical-officers/the-evolution-of-the-chief-medical-officer.

40 Ibid.

41 Christopher G. Myers, Daniel Polsky, and Sanjay Desai, "The Growing Role of Chief Medical Officers in Major Corporations," *JAMA Health Forum*, July 22, 2022, https://jamanetwork.com/journals/jama-health-forum/fullarticle/27944537.

42 American Hospital Association, op. cit.

43 Ibid.

44 Francesca Mathewes, "The evolution of the chief medical officer," *Becker's Physician Leadership*, June 24, 2025, https://www.beckersphysicianleadership.com/chief-medical-officers/the-evolution-of-the-chief-medical-officer.

45 Interview with Allen Verrill, July 22, 2025.

46 Interview with Ken Lukhard, June 18, 2025.

47 Christopher G. Myers, Daniel Polsky, and Sanjay Desai, op. cit.

48 Christopher G. Myers, Daniel Polsky, and Sanjay Desai, op. cit.

49 Rick Scott, email message to author.

50 Christopher G. Myers, Daniel Polsky, and Sanjay Desai, op. cit.

51 T. Quince, M. Abbas, S. Murugesu, F. Crawley, S. Hyde, D. Wood et. al., "Leadership and Management in the Undergraduate Medical Curriculum: A Qualitative Study of Students' Attitudes and Opinions at One UK Medical School," *BMJ Open* 4, e005350, 2014, doi:10.1136/bmjopen-2014-005353.

52 "Leadership Development," AAMC, accessed March 17, 2026, https://www.aamc.org/learn-network/leadership-development.

53 American Hospital Association, op. cit.

54 Ibid.

55 "Leadership Development," AAMC, accessed March 17, 2026, https://www.aamc.org/learn-network/leadership-development.

56 Brendan Murphy, "Leadership 101: What medical students need to know," AMA, July 28, 2025, https://www.ama-assn.org/education/changemeded-initiative/leadership-101-what-medical-students-need-know.

57 Meyers et al.

58 David Nash, "Who's at the Helm? The Evolving Role of the Physician Executive," *MedPage Today*, January 3, 2023, https:/www.medpagetoday.com/opinion/focos-on-policy/102480.

59 Peter B. Angood, "Physician Leadership: More Valuable Than Ever—A White Paper from the American Association for Physician Leadership," September 2022, page 1, www.physicianleaders.org/articles/doi/10.55834.wp.9897031832.

60 E. V. Stagg, "Hospitals Ramp Up Training for Physician Leadership Roles," *American Medical News*, February 23, 2012.

61 Angood, page 1.

62 Ibid., page 2.

63 Ibid.

64 Ibid., page 4.

65 Ibid., page 4.

66 Ibid., page 4.

67 Francesca Mathewes, "Physicians' journey back to the C-suite," *Becker's Physician Leadership*, August 5, 2025, www.beckersphysicianleadership.com/leadership/physicians-journey-back-to-the-C-suite/.

68 Mariah Taylor, "The shrinking physician leadership pipeline," *Becker's Hospital Review*, June 6, 2025, https://www.beckershospitalreview.com/quality/hospital-physician-relationships/the-shrinking-physician-leadership-pipeline/.

69 Ibid.

70 Ibid.

71 Angood, page 15.

72 Angood, page 4.

73 Angood, page 15.

74 Angood, page 3.

75 Angood, page 3.

76 Angood, page 12.

77 Angood, page 13.

78 Michael J. Menen, "The Role of the CMO," *American Association of Physician Leadership*, January 20, 2025, https://www.physicianleaders.org/articles/role-of-the-CMO.

79 Ibid.

80 Angood, page 5.

81 Interview with Elise MacCarroll Wright, September 23, 2025.

82 Francesca Mathewes, "What should physician leadership look like?" *Becker's Physician Leadership*, July 17, 2025, https://www.beckersphysicianleadership.com/leadership/what-should-physician-leadership-look-like.

83 Angood, page 3.

84 Angood, pages 15–16.

85 Eric Sabol, "Seven Characteristics that Define a Physician Leader," *American Association of Physician Leadership*, April 27, 2018, https://www.physician leaders.org/seven-characteristics-that-define-a-physician-leader.

86 Mathewes, "What should physician leadership look like?" op. cit.

87 Ibid.

88 Angood, page 3.

89 Angood, page 7.

90 Angood, pages 1–2.

91 Physician, email message to author. The name of the interviewee is withheld by mutual agreement.

92 Angood, page 5.

93 Sara Berg, "5 reasons physicians are less likely to seek support," July 30, 2018. https://www.ama-assn.org/practice-management/physician-health/5-reasons-physicians-are-less-likely-seek-support.

94 Ibid.

95 Angood, page 9.

96 Andrew Proulx, "Physician Suicide: Suicide Rates Among HCPs in the US," *Psychiatry Advisor*, September 12, 2025, https://www.psychiatryadvisor.com/feature/physician-suicide.

97 Ibid.

98 Ibid.

99 Hirsh Makhija, Judy E. Davidson, Kelly C. Lee et al., "National Incidence of Physician Suicide and Associated Features," *JAMA Psychiatry*, February 26, 2025, https://jamanetwork.com/journals/jamapsychiatry/fullarticle/2830401?guestAccessKey=5b54efa5-f490-4c36-9879-6e5bd722985e.

100 Ibid.

101 "COVID-19's Impact on Physician Wellbeing," survey completed in September 2020 by the Physicians Foundation, https://physiciansfoundation.org/research/the-physicians-foundation-2020-physician-survey-part-2/.

102 Ibid.

103 Xiaoming Zhang et. al., “Physician Workforce in the United States of America: forecasting nationwide shortages,” *Human Resource Health*, February 6, 2020, https://pmc.nchi.hlm.nih.gov/articles/PMC7006215.

104 “Physician Workforce: Projections, 2020–2035,” National Center for Health Workforce Analysis, November 2022, https://bhw.hrsa.gov/sites/default/files/bureau-health-workforce/Physicians-Projections-Factsheet.pdf.

105 Advanced Practice Partners LLC is a national group of physicians who serve as physician collaborators to nurse practitioners, physician assistants, and nurses seeking clinical supervision.

106 Interview with CFO, May 14, 2025. The name of the interviewee is withheld by mutual agreement.

107 “Quality of care,” World Health Organization, accessed March 17, 2026, https://www.who.int/health-topics/quality-of-care/#tab=tab_1.

108 “The Value of Dyads for Improved Healthcare Leadership,” MDA Leadership, 2024, https://mdaleadership.com/resources/white-papers/the-value-of-dyads-for-improved-healthcare-leadership/.

109 Ibid.

110 Ibid.

111 Adapted from “Ultimate Guide to the National Patient Safety Goals 2025 (NPSGs),” American Data Network, May 2, 2025, https://www.americandatanetwork.com/patient-safety/national-patient-safety-goals-2025/.

112 Ibid.

113 Ibid.

114 Ibid.

115 "Ultimate Guide to the National Patient Safety Goals 2025 (NPSGs)," op. cit.

116 "Effective: good," CareQuality Commission, last updated May 12, 2022, https://www.cqc.org.uk/guidance-providers/healthcare/effective-good.

117 Alisa Khan, M. W. Ramotar, C. P. Landrigan, "Does a Patient-and Family-Centered Hospital Communications Program Reduce Medical Errors?" Patient-Centered Outcomes Research Institute (PCORI), 2019, https://www.pcori.org/research-results/2013/does-patient-and-family-centered-hospital-communications-program-reduce-medical-errors.

118 "Engagement in Research," PCORI, accessed March 18, 2026, https://www.pcori.org/funding-opportunities/what-we-mean-engagement.

119 "Engaging Patient and Family Advisors in Research," Institute for Patient- and Family-Centered Care, accessed March 17, 2026, https://www.ipfcc.org/bestpractices/sustainable-partnerships/engaging/index html.

120 "OECD Health Policy Studies," Organisation for Economic Co-operation and Development, accessed March 18, 2026, https://www.oecd.org/en/publications/oecd-health-policy-studies_2074319x.html.

121 Based on Dean McConnell, JD, COPIC Deputy General Counsel, "What Every Facility Should Know About Patient Complaints and Grievances," https://www.copic.com/wp-content/uploads/2024/12/what-every-patient-advocate-must-know-about-patient-complaints-and-grievances.pdf.

122 "Grievances," Centers for Medicare and Medicaid Services, last modified September 10, 2024, https://www.cms.gov/medicare/appeals-grievances/managed-care/grievances.

123 Based on information in “Disclosure and Discussion of Adverse Events,” ACOG Clinical, December 2016, https://www.acog.org/clinical/clinical-guidance/committee-opinion/articles/2016/12/disclosure-and-discussion-of-adverse-events.

124 Debbie LaValley, “Adverse Events Disclosure,” CRICO, September 12, 2016, https://rmf.harvard.edu/Risk-Prevention-and-Education/Guidelines-and-Algorithms-Catalog-Page/Guidelines-Algorithms/2009/Guidelines-for-Disclosure.

125 For additional counsel and guidance, see the Agency for Healthcare Research and Quality’s Module 5: Response and Disclosure, content last reviewed August 2022, https://www.ahrq.gov/patient-safety/settings/hospital/candor/modules/guide5/notes.html.

126 Don Jernigan, *The Hidden Power of Relentless Stewardship* (Rosetta Books, 2016), 33.

127 Jernigan, 34.

128 Jernigan, 34, 35.

129 Jernigan, 35.

130 Benedikt Langenberger, Christopher Worsham, and Pascal Geldsetzer, “The Effect of Length of Stay in Hospital on Patients’ Health Outcomes,” PubMed, National Library of Medicine, December 2024. https://pmc.ncbi.nlm.nih.gov/articles/PMC11643150.

131 JAMA, July 4, 2017; 318; (1): 93-94.

132 Kari A. Phillips, Naykky Singh Ospina, Victor M. Montori, “Physicians Interrupting Patients, ” *Journal of General Internal Medicine* 34(10): 1965, August 6, 2019, doi.org/10.1007/s11606-019-05247-5.

133 Ibid.

134 Ibid.

135 Peter B. Angood, "Physician Leadership: More Valuable Than Ever—A White Paper from the American Association for Physician Leadership," September 2022, www.physicianleaders.org/articles/doi/10.55834.wp.9897031832.

136 Ibid., page 8.

137 Ibid., page 8.

138 Interview with chief nursing officer, June 6, 2025. The name of the interviewee is withheld by mutual agreement.

139 "The Value of Dyads for Improved Healthcare Leadership," MDA Leadership, 2024, https://mdaleadership.com/resources/white-papers/the-value-of-dyads-for-improved-healthcare-leadership/.

140 Interview with director of quality and patient safety, June 9, 2025. The name of the interviewee is withheld by mutual agreement.

141 "well-being," Merriam-Webster, accessed March 17, 2026, https://www.merriam-webster.com/dictionary/well-being.

142 Peter B. Angood, "Physician Leadership: More Valuable Than Ever—A White Paper from the American Association for Physician Leadership," September 2022, www.physicianleaders.org/articles/doi/10.55834.wp.9897031832.

143 Mariah Taylor, "Split physician roles in action: A guide from AMCs," *Becker's Clinical Leadership*, July 25, 2025, https://www.beckershospitalreview.com/quality/hospital-physician-relationships/split-physician-in-action-a-guide-from-amcs/.

144 Angood, op. cit.

145 Jeffrey B. Kramer, MD, in "Doctors Extending Their Education: *Why an MBA? Is It a Degree of Success?*" National Library of Medicine, https://pme.ncbi.hlm.nih.gov/articles/PMC6179538/.

146 Adrian J. Delaney III, in "Doctors Extending Their Education: *Why an MBA? Is It a Degree of Success?*" National Library of Medicine, https://pme.ncbi.hlm.nih.gov/articles/PMC6179538/.

147 Interview with OB/GYN, September 15, 2025. The name of the interviewee is withheld by mutual agreement.

148 "The Costs of Caring: Challenges Facing America's Hospitals in 2025," American Hospital Association, accessed April 2025, https://www.aha.org/costsofcaring.

149 Brenda Goodman, "Insurer and cancer center reach agreement in contract dispute that left thousands of patients in limbo," *CNN*, July 1, 2025, https://www.cnn.com/2025/07/01/health/united-healthcare-memorial-sloan-kettering-contract-cancer.

150 "Duke Health and Aetna Contract Negotiation," DukeHealth, accessed March 17, 2026, https://www.dukehealth.org/aetna.

151 Bram Sable-Smith, "When Hospitals and Insurers Fight, Patients Get Caught in the Middle," *KFF Health News*, September 2, 2025, https://kffhealthnews.org/news/article/hospitals-insurers-contract-dispute-patients-coverage-in-limbo/.

152 "The No Suprises Act's Continuity of Care, Provider Directory, and Public Disclosure Requirements," Centers for Medicare and Medicaid Services, accessed March 17, 2026, https://www.cms.gov/files/document/a274577-1b-training-2nsa-disclosure-continuity-care-directoriesfinal-508.pdf.

153 Don Jernigan, *The Hidden Power of Relentless Stewardship* (Rosetta Books, 2016), 32–33.

154 Bismarck C. Odei, Crystal Seldon, and Melanie Fernandez et al., "Representation of Women in the Leadership Structure of the US Health Care System," Jama Netw Open, https://pmc.ncbi.nlm.nih.gov/articles/PMC8630566/#zld210261r4.

155 Bismarck C. Odei, Crystal Seldon, and Melanie Fernandez et al., "Representation of Women in the Leadership Structure of the US Health Care System," JAMA Netw Open 4(11):e2136358, November 29, 2021, doi: 10.1001/jamanetworkopen.2021.36358.

156 Adapted from Steve Fiorillo, "History of Women in Medicine," *Medical Professionals Reference*, March 7, 2025, https://www.empr.com/features/history-of-women-in-medicine.

www.ingramcontent.com/pod-product-compliance
Lightning Source LLC
LaVergne TN
LVHW100608120926
847902LV00001B/3